Atlas of the Human Brain

ATLAS OF THE HUMAN BRAIN

LOTHAR JENNES, Ph.D.
Associate Professor of Anatomy and Neurobiology
University of Kentucky College of Medicine
Lexington, Kentucky

HAROLD H. TRAURIG, Ph.D.
Professor of Anatomy and Neurobiology
University of Kentucky College of Medicine
Lexington, Kentucky

P. MICHAEL CONN, Ph.D.
Associate Provost for Extended Campus
and Biotechnology Development
Professor of Pharmacology
Oregon Health Sciences University
Portland, Oregon
Associate Director for Research and Development
Oregon Regional Primate Research Center
Beaverton, Oregon

J. B. LIPPINCOTT COMPANY
Philadelphia

Acquisitions Editor: Richard Winters
Project Editor: Ellen M. Campbell
Indexer: Ann Blum
Designer: Doug Smock
Cover Designer: Louis Fuiano
Production Manager: Caren Erlichman
Senior Production Coordinator: Kevin P. Johnson
Compositor: Compset, Inc.
Printer/Binder: Arcata Graphics/Kingsport

6 5 4 3 2 1

Library of Congress Cataloging–in–Publications Data

Jennes, Lothar
    Atlas of the human brain / Lothar Jennes, Harold H. Traurig,
P. Michael Conn.
      p. cm.
    Includes index.
    ISBN 0–397–51277–5
    1. Brain—Atlases.   2. Neuroanatomy—Atlases.   3. Central nervous
system—Atlases.   I. Traurig, Harold H.   II. Conn, P. Michael.
III. Title.
    [DNLM: 1. Brain—anatomy & histology—atlases.   2. Spinal Cord—
anatomy & histology—atlases.   3. Peripheral Nervous System—
anatomy & histology—atlases.   WL 17 J54a 1995]
    QM455, J46   1995
    611′.81′0222—dc20
    DNLM/DLC
    for Library of Congress   94–13093
                                    CIP

♾ This Paper Meets the Requirements of ANSI/NISO Z39.48–1992
(Permanence of Paper).

The authors and publishers have exerted every effort to ensure that drug
selection and dosage set forth in this text are in accord with current
recommendations and practice at the time of publication. However, in view of
ongoing research, changes in government regulations, and the constant flow
of information relating to drug therapy and drug reactions, the reader is
urged to check the package insert for each drug for any change in indications
and dosage and for added warnings and precautions. This is particularly
important when the recommended agent is a new or infrequently employed
drug.

Preface

When we were asked to put together a neuroanatomy atlas, our initial response was why, since there are already several good atlases available. After discussions with teachers, clinicians, and students, however, we felt that there is indeed a need for a comprehensive atlas which covers contemporary neuroanatomy along with traditional material. The *Atlas of the Human Brain* was therefore designed to include not only the traditional neuroanatomy of the central nervous system, but also extensive chapters on modern diagnostic approaches, such as high-speed and resolution angiograms and CT scans and MRIs of normative and pathological nervous tissue. It is essential for today's student to be thoroughly familiar with these contemporary imaging techniques.

The atlas begins with a traditional presentation of the gross anatomy of the brain (Chapter 1), followed by a coronal series of thick sections through the brain which shows the major structures of the central nervous system (Chapter 2). More detailed information is then shown in series of coronal (Chapter 3) and horizontal (Chapter 4) Weigert-stained sections, as well as in higher magnification series through the brain stem (Chapter 5), and select regions of the spinal cord (Chapter 6). The blood supply of the brain is presented with extensive angiograms, including a time-course series which demonstrates the passage of blood through the arterial, capillary and venous phases, as well as ex-amples of pathological conditions (Chapter 7). The anatomy of the brain and spinal cord, including the cere-broventricular system and the blood supply, can then be studied in an integrated fashion with several series of CT and MRI scans. These scans were taken with different enhancement settings in order to show gray or white matter, cerebrospinal fluid, or blood (Chapter 8). An extensive description of various frequent pathological conditions of the brain and spinal cord follows (Chapter 9). Detailed chapters on the light and electron microscopic features of the central and peripheral nervous system, including eye, ear, and sensory nerve endings (Chapters 10–12), conclude the atlas.

We would like to take this opportunity to thank many people who contributed to this atlas. Drs. Bruce Maley, John Porter, Karin Sikora-VanMeter, and Raymond Papka are acknowledged for providing the electron mi-crographs, as is Dr. Donald Buxton for allowing us to use his sections of muscle spindles and Dr. Stephen Scheff for sections of brains with Alzheimer's disease. We also thank Mrs. Mary Gail Engle for the photo-graphic work of the electron micrographs, and Mr. Mo-hamad Haleem, Curator of the Yakovlev Collection, for his help with the selection of the Weigert-stained brain series, as well as the Armed Forces Institute of Pathol-ogy for making this resource available to us. Thanks also to the artistic and editorial staff at Lippincott for their help and counsel.

Contents

Atlas of the Human Brain

Atlas of the Human Brain, by Lothar Jennes, Harold H. Traurig, and P. Michael Conn. J. B. Lippincott Company, Philadelphia, © 1995.

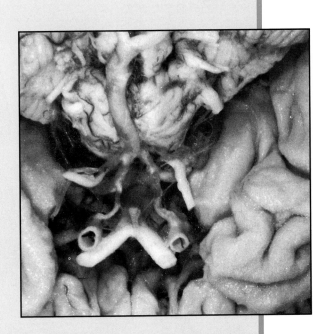

Gross Anatomy of the Brain

c h a p t e r 1

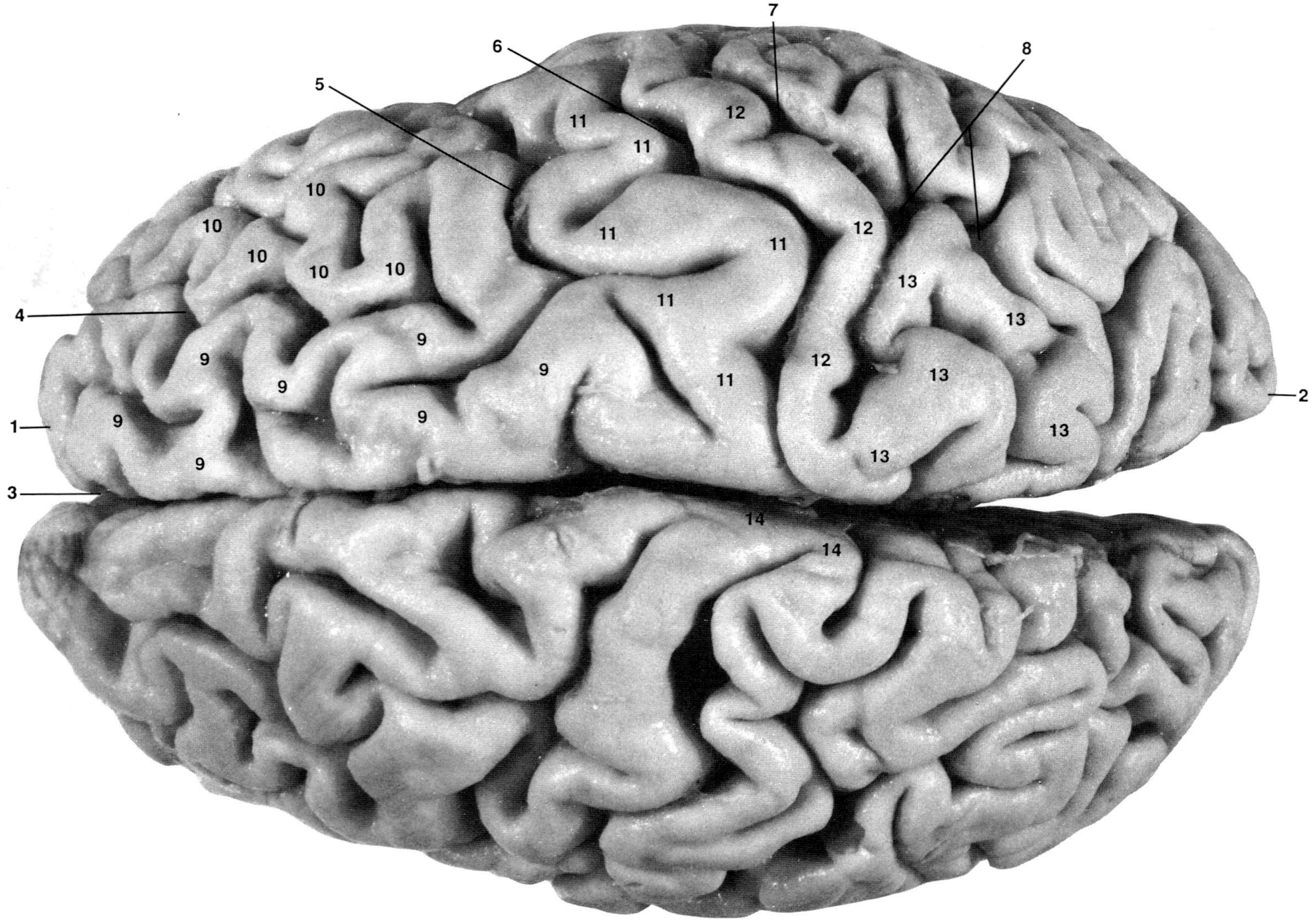

Gross Anatomy of the Brain

1. Frontal pole
2. Occipital pole
3. Interhemispheric fissure
4. Superior frontal sulcus
5. Precentral sulcus
6. Central sulcus
7. Posterior central sulcus
8. Interparietal sulcus
9. Superior frontal gyrus
10. Middle frontal gyrus
11. Precentral gyrus
12. Postcentral gyrus
13. Superior parietal lobule
14. Paracentral lobule

FIGURE 1-1.
Superior surface of the cerebral hemispheres.

Gross Anatomy of the Brain

1. Frontal pole
2. Occipital pole
3. Interhemispheric fissure
4. Superior frontal sulcus
5. Precentral sulcus
6. Central sulcus
7. Postcentral sulcus
8. Interparietal sulcus
9. Superior frontal gyrus
10. Middle frontal gyrus
11. Precentral gyrus
12. Postcentral gyrus
13. Superior parietal lobule
15. Inferior frontal gyrus, pars triangularis
16. Inferior frontal gyrus, pars orbitalis
17. Inferior frontal gyrus, pars opercularis
18. Lateral fissure
19. Temporal pole
20. Superior temporal gyrus
21. Middle temporal gyrus
22. Superior temporal sulcus
23. Supramarginal gyrus
24. Angular gyrus
25. Cerebellum

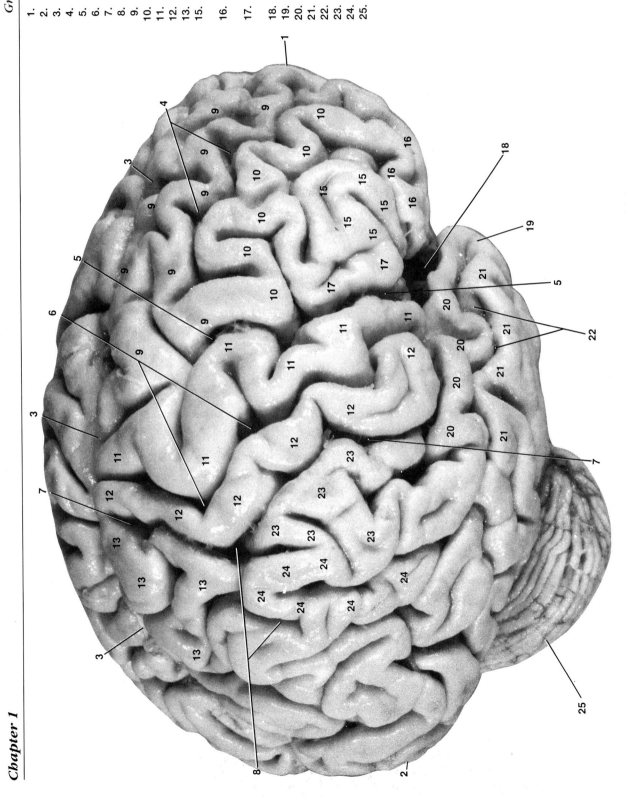

FIGURE 1-2.
Lateral view of the right hemisphere.

Gross Anatomy of the Brain

1. Frontal pole
2. Occipital pole
3. Interhemispheric fissure
4. Superior frontal sulcus
5. Precentral sulcus
6. Central sulcus
7. Postcentral sulcus
8. Interparietal sulcus
9. Superior frontal gyrus
10. Middle frontal gyrus
11. Precentral gyrus
12. Postcentral gyrus
15. Inferior frontal gyrus, pars triangularis
16. Inferior frontal gyrus, pars orbitalis
17. Inferior frontal gyrus, pars opercularis
18. Lateral fissure
19. Temporal pole
20. Superior temporal gyrus
21. Middle temporal gyrus
22. Superior temporal sulcus
23. Supramarginal gyrus
24. Angular gyrus
25. Cerebellum
26. Inferior frontal sulcus

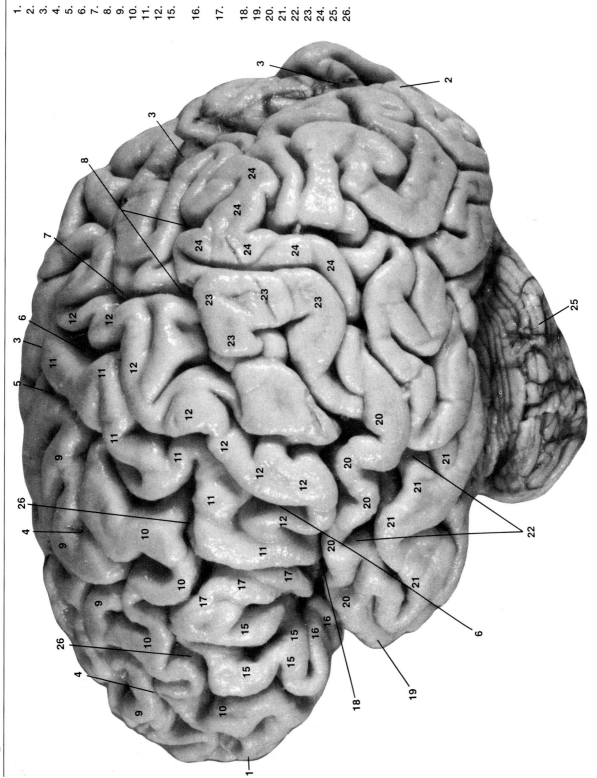

FIGURE 1-3.
Lateral view of the left hemisphere which is dominant in right-handed individuals.

Gross Anatomy of the Brain

1. Frontal pole
2. Occipital pole
3. Interhemispheric fissure
16. Inferior frontal gyrus, pars orbitalis
19. Temporal pole
21. Middle temporal gyrus
25. Cerebellum
27. Inferior temporal gyrus
28. Parahippocampal gyrus
29. Uncus
30. Straight gyrus
31. Olfactory bulb
32. Olfactory sulcus
33. Orbital gyri
34. Olfactory tract
35. Olfactory trigone
36. Optic nerve
37. Infundibulum
38. Collateral sulcus
39. Basilar artery
40. Pons (middle cerebellar peduncle)
41. Flocculus
42. Vertebral artery
43. Medulla
44. Branches of posterior inferior cerebellar artery

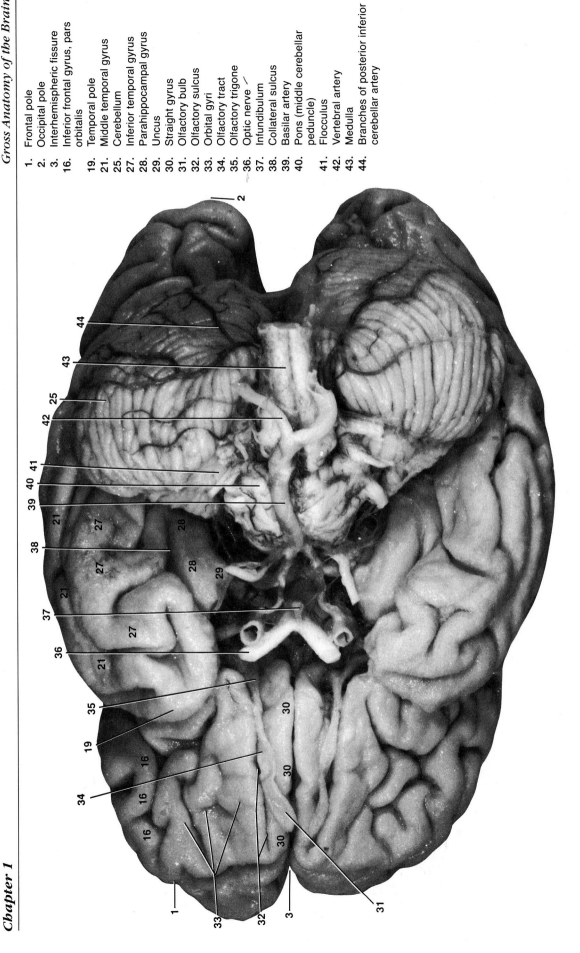

FIGURE 1-4.
Inferior surface of the brain.

Gross Anatomy of the Brain

27. Inferior temporal gyrus
28. Parahippocampal gyrus
29. Uncus
30. Straight gyrus
34. Olfactory tract
35. Olfactory trigone
36. Optic nerve
39. Basilar artery
42. Vertebral artery
45. Optic chiasm
46. Internal carotid artery
47. Posterior communicating artery
48. Oculomotor nerve (III)
49. Posterior cerebral artery
50. Interpeduncular fossa (cistern)
51. Superior cerebellar artery
52. Roots of trigeminal nerve (V)
53. Vestibular-cochlear (VIII) and facial nerve (VII)
54. Choroid plexus
55. Tonsils of cerebellum
56. Middle cerebral artery
57. Anterior perforated substance
58. Posterior inferior cerebellar artery

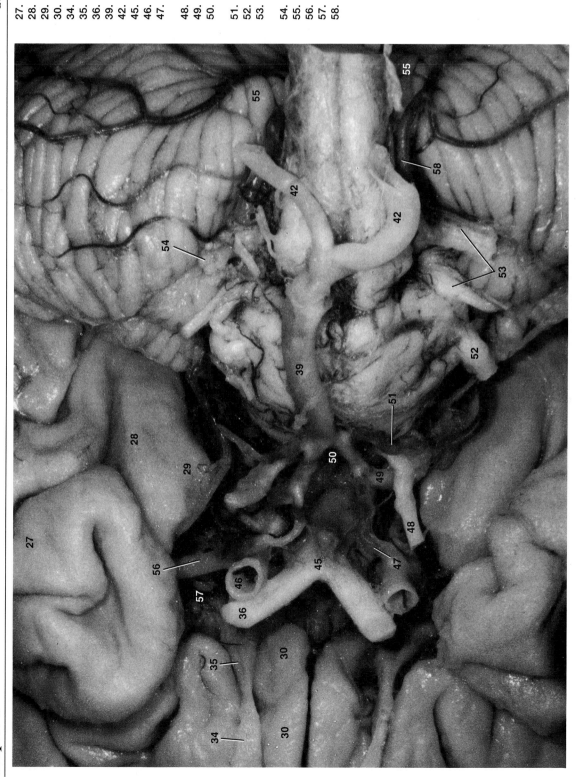

FIGURE 1-5.
Inferior surface of the brain at higher magnification.

Gross Anatomy of the Brain

1. Frontal pole
2. Occipital pole
3. Temporal pole
4. Precentral gyrus ⎱ Paracentral
5. Postcentral gyrus ⎰ gyrus
6. Cingulate gyrus
7. Cingulate sulcus
8. Central sulcus
9. Superior frontal gyrus
10. Calcarine sulcus
11. Cuneus
12. Precuneus
13. Lingual gyrus
14. Parieto-occipital sulcus
15. Genu of corpus callosum
16. Body of corpus callosum
17. Splenium of corpus callosum
18. Septum pellucidum
19. Parolfactory gyrus (septum)
20. Gyrus rectus
21. Hypothalamus and third ventricle
22. Mammillary body
23. Optic chiasm
24. Anterior commissure
25. Massa intermedia
26. Thalamus and third ventricle
27. Body of lateral ventricle
28. Interventricular foramen of Monro
29. Body of Fornix
30. Pineal
31. Posterior commissure
32. Superior colliculus
33. Inferior colliculus
34. Cerebral aqueduct
35. Anterior medullary velum
36. Fourth ventricle
37. Posterior medullary velum and choroid plexus
38. Cerebellum (vermis)
39. Midbrain
40. Interpeduncular cistern
41. Pons
42. Medulla

7

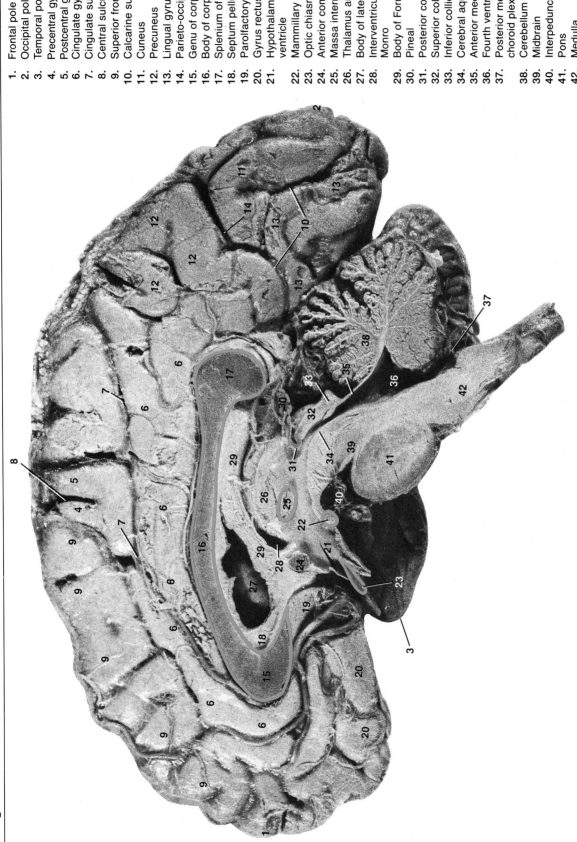

FIGURE 1-6.
Medial surface of the right hemisphere.

1. Rostrum of corpus callosum
2. Genu of corpus callosum
3. Body of corpus callosum
4. Splenium of corpus callosum
5. Septum pellucidum
6. Body of lateral ventricle
7. Body of fornix
8. Column of fornix
9. Interventricular foramen of Monro
10. Thalamus
11. Massa intermedia
12. Hypothalamic sulcus
13. Third ventricle covering the hypothalamus
14. Anterior commissure
15. Lamina terminalis
16. Optic chiasm
17. Optic nerve
18. Infundibular recess of third ventricle
19. Mammillary body
20. Interpeduncular cistern
21. Midbrain
22. Pons
23. Medulla
24. Posterior medullary velum
25. Fourth ventricle
26. Anterior medullary velum
27. Inferior colliculus
28. Superior colliculus
29. Posterior commissure
30. Quadrigeminal cistern
31. Habenula
32. Pineal
33. Stria medullaris
34. Cingulate gyrus

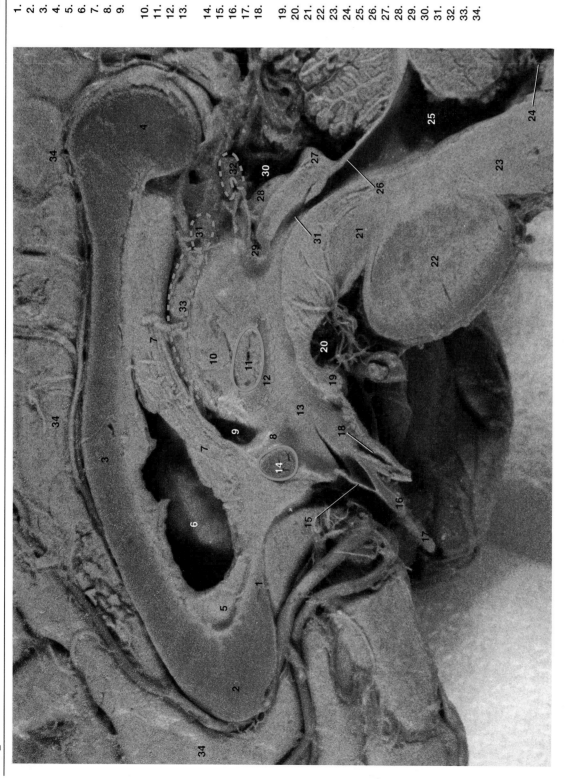

FIGURE 1-7.

Higher magnification of midsagittal section of a brain showing the diencephalon and brainstem.

1. Frontal operculum
2. Parietal operculum
3. Transverse gyri of Heschl
4. Insular cortex
5. Superior temporal gyrus
6. Middle temporal gyrus
7. Frontal pole
8. Occipital pole

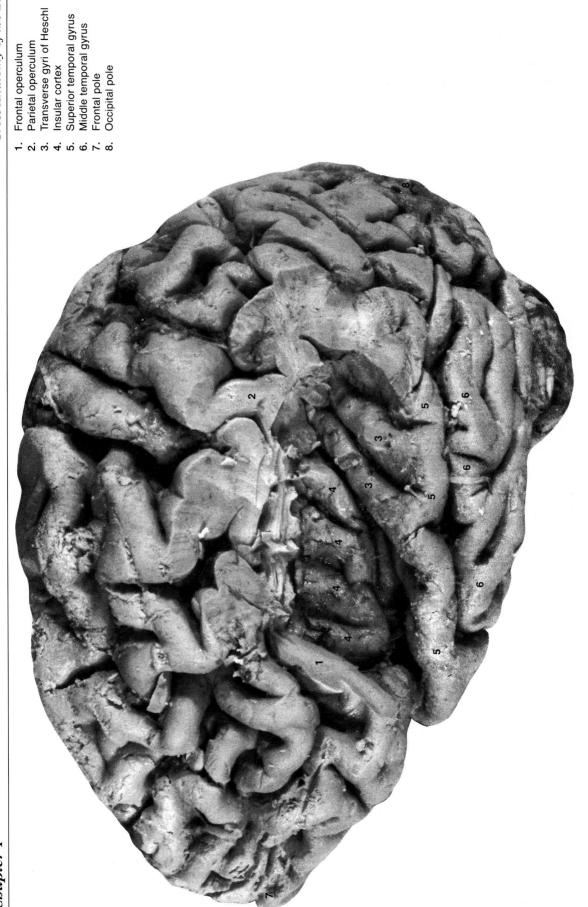

FIGURE 1-8.
Lateral view of the left hemisphere with the frontal (1) and parietal (2) operculum removed revealing the transverse gyri of Heschl (3; auditory cortex and areas 41 and 42 of Brodmann). The cortex of the insula (4) lies deep to the lateral fissure.

Gross Anatomy of the Brain

1. Spinal cord
2. Tonsil of cerebellum
3. Nodulus of cerebellum
4. Vertebral artery
5. Basilar artery
6. Cisterna magna
7. Fourth ventricle

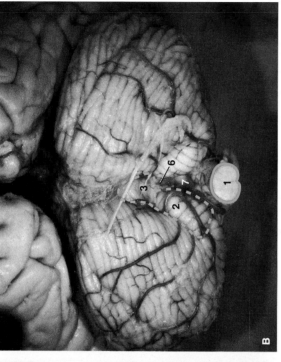

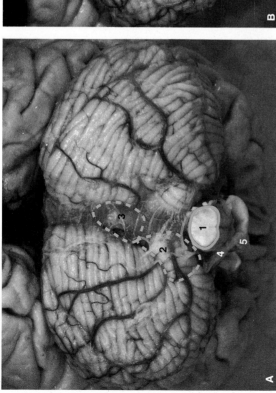

FIGURE 1-9.

Inferior view of the cerebellum showing the location of the cisterna magna (**A**) before and (**B**) after removal of the meninges.

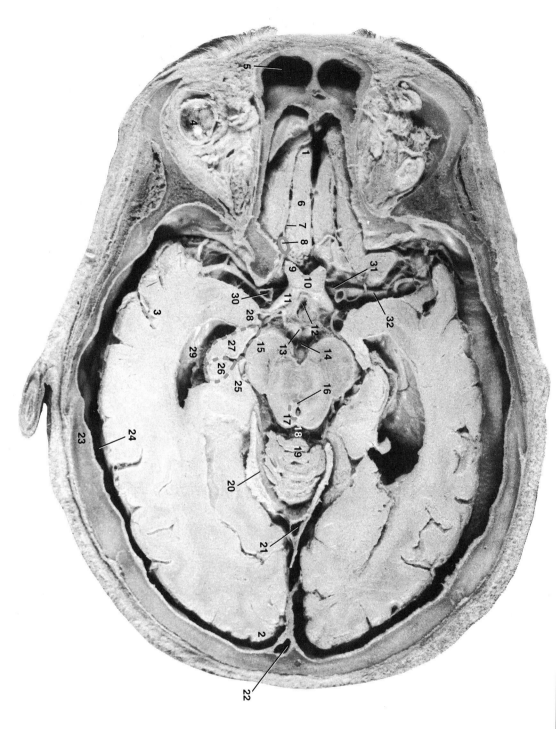

FIGURE 1-10.
Horizontal section through the head at the level of the hypothalamus (inferior view).

1. Frontal pole
2. Occipital pole
3. Temporal lobe
4. Globe in orbit
5. Frontal sinus
6. Gyrus rectus
7. Olfactory sulcus
8. Olfactory tract
9. Optic nerve
10. Optic chiasm
11. Optic tract
12. Third ventricle
13. Mammillary body
14. Interpeduncular cistern
15. Cerebral peduncle
16. Periaqueductal gray
17. Superior colliculus
18. Quadrigeminal cistern
19. Superior vermis of cerebellum
20. Tentorium cerebelli
21. Straight sinus
22. Superior sagittal sinus
23. Parietal bone
24. Subdural space
25. Parahippocampal gyrus
26. Hippocampus
27. Subiculum
28. Uncus and amygdala
29. Inferior horn of lateral ventricle
30. Internal carotid artery
31. Anterior cerebral artery
32. Middle cerebral artery

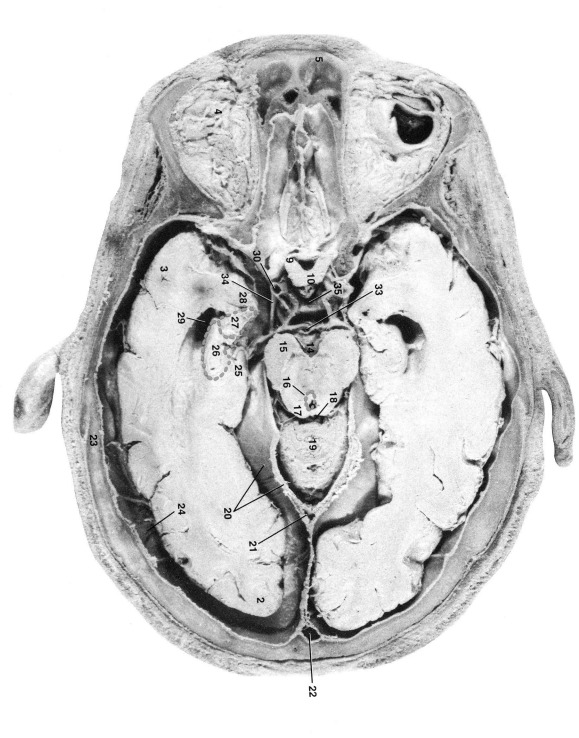

FIGURE 1-11.
Horizontal section through the head at the level of the dorsal sella turcica (superior view).

2. Occipital pole
3. Temporal lobe
4. Globe in orbit
5. Frontal sinus
9. Optic nerve
10. Optic chiasm
14. Interpeduncular cistern
15. Cerebral peduncle
16. Periaqueductal gray
17. Superior colliculus
18. Quadrigeminal cistern
19. Superior vermis of cerebellum
20. Tentorium cerebelli
21. Straight sinus
22. Superior sagittal sinus
23. Parietal bone
24. Subdural space
25. Parahippocampal gyrus
26. Hippocampus
27. Subiculum
28. Uncus and amygdala
29. Inferior horn of lateral
    ventricle
30. Internal carotid artery
33. Basilar artery
34. Posterior communicating
    artery
35. Sella turcica.

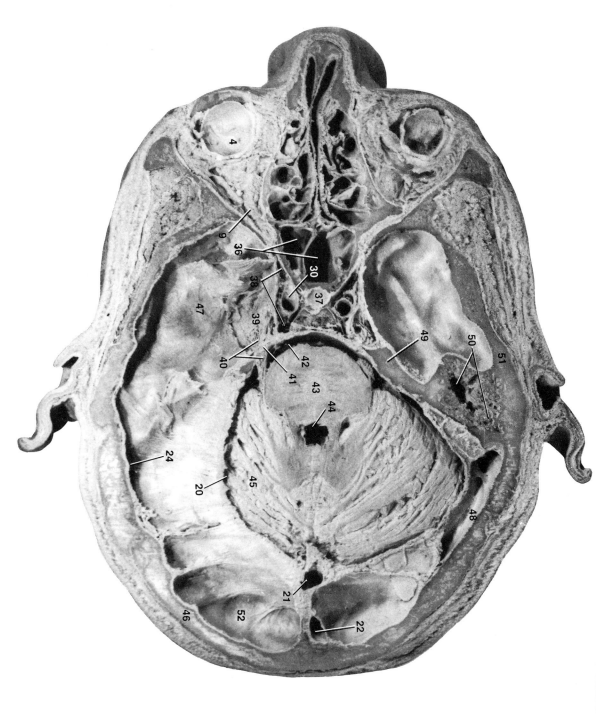

FIGURE 1-12.
Horizontal section through the head at the level of the trigeminal ganglion (superior view).

4. Globe in orbit
9. Optic nerve
20. Tentorium cerebelli
21. Straight sinus
22. Superior sagittal sinus
24. Subdural space
30. Internal carotid artery
36. Nasal pharynx
37. Hypophysis in sella turcica
38. Cavernous sinus
39. Trigeminal ganglion
40. Trigeminal nerve
41. Superior petrosal sinus
42. Pontine cistern
43. Pons
44. Fourth ventricle
45. Lateral hemisphere of cerebellum
46. Occipital bone
47. Middle cranial fossa (position of temporal lobe)
48. Lateral sinus
49. Petrous ridge of temporal bone
50. Labyrinth and mastoid air cells
51. Squamous portion of temporal bone
52. Supratentorial space (position of occipital lobe)

Coronal Slices of the Brain

(Unstained)

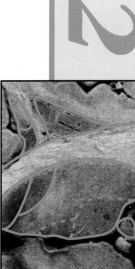

Atlas of the Human Brain, by Lothar Jennes,
Harold H. Traurig, and P. Michael Conn.
J. B. Lippincott Company, Philadelphia, © 1995.

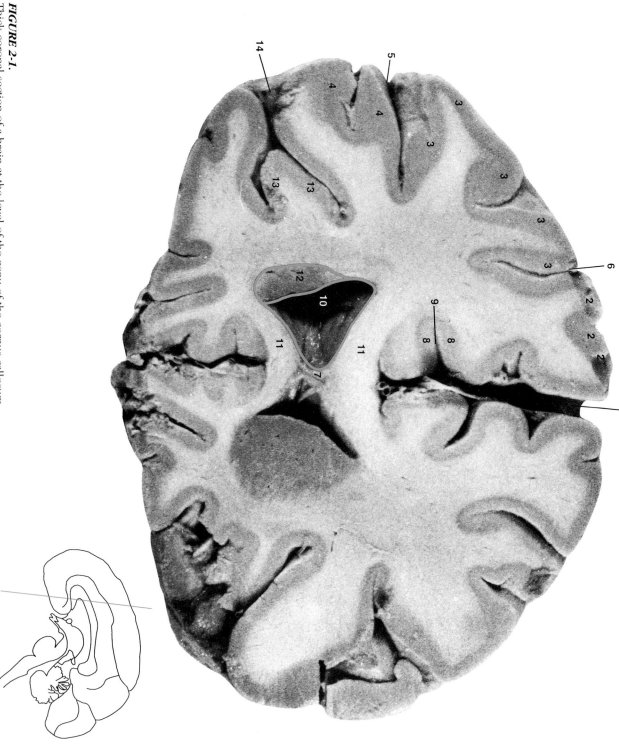

FIGURE 2-1.
Thick coronal section of a brain at the level of the genu of the corpus callosum.

1. Interhemispheric fissure
2. Superior frontal gyrus
3. Middle frontal gyrus
4. Inferior frontal gyrus
5. Inferior frontal sulcus
6. Superior frontal sulcus
7. Septum pellucidum
8. Cingulate gyrus
9. Cingulate sulcus
10. Anterior horn of lateral ventricle
11. Genu of corpus callosum
12. Head of caudate nucleus
13. Insula
14. Lateral sulcus (Sylvian fissure)

Coronal Slices of the Brain (Unstained)

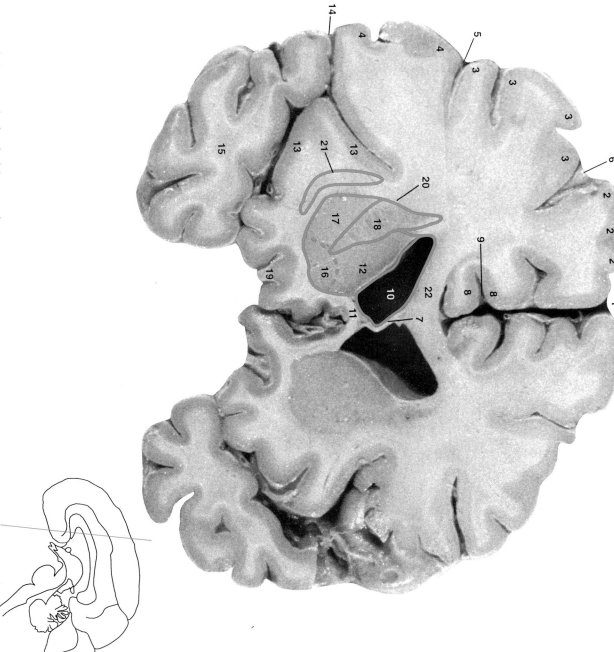

FIGURE 2-2.
Thick coronal section of a brain at the level of the rostral striatum.

1. Interhemispheric fissure
2. Superior frontal gyrus
3. Middle frontal gyrus
4. Inferior frontal gyrus
5. Inferior frontal sulcus
6. Superior frontal sulcus
7. Septum pellucidum
8. Cingulate gyrus
9. Cingulate sulcus
10. Anterior horn of lateral ventricle
11.
12. Head of caudate nucleus
13. Insula
14. Lateral sulcus (Sylvian fissure)
15. Temporal lobe
16. Nucleus accumbens
17. Putamen
18. Anterior limb of internal capsule
19. Olfactory tract
20. External capsule
21. Claustrum
22. Body of corpus callosum

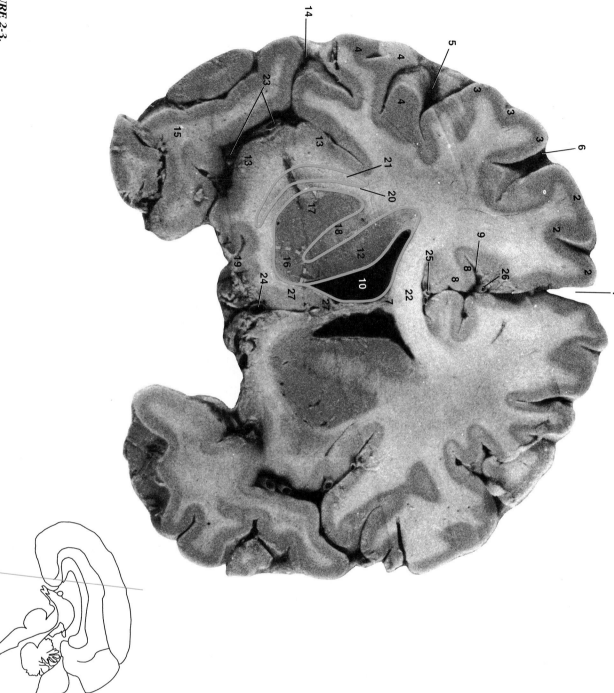

FIGURE 2-3.
Thick coronal section of a brain just rostral to the optic chiasm.

1. Interhemispheric fissure
2. Superior frontal gyrus
3. Middle frontal gyrus
4. Inferior frontal gyrus
5. Inferior frontal sulcus
6. Superior frontal sulcus
7. Septum pellucidum
8. Cingulate gyrus
9. Cingulate sulcus
10. Anterior horn of lateral ventricle
11. Head of caudate nucleus
12. Head of caudate nucleus
13. Insula
14. Lateral sulcus (Sylvian fissure)
15. Temporal lobe
16. Nucleus accumbens
17. Putamen
18. Anterior limb of internal capsule
19. Olfactory tract
20. External capsule
21. Claustrum
22. Body of corpus callosum
23. Sylvian branches of middle cerebral artery
24. Anterior cerebral artery
25. Pericallosal branch of anterior cerebral artery
26. Calloso-marginal branch of anterior cerebral artery
27. Septum (parolfactory gyrus)

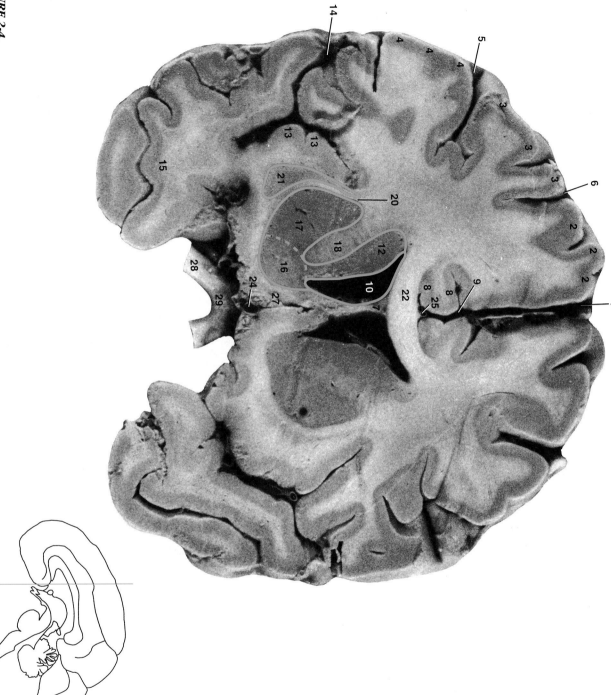

FIGURE 2-4.
Thick coronal section of a brain at the level of the optic chiasm.

1. Interhemispheric fissure
2. Superior frontal gyrus
3. Middle frontal gyrus
4. Inferior frontal gyrus
5. Inferior frontal sulcus
6. Superior frontal sulcus
7. Septum pellucidum
8. Cingulate gyrus
9. Cingulate sulcus
10. Anterior horn of lateral ventricle
12. Head of caudate nucleus
13. Insula
14. Lateral sulcus (Sylvian fissure)
15. Temporal lobe
16. Nucleus accumbens
17. Putamen
18. Anterior limb of internal capsule
20. External capsule
21. Claustrum
22. Body of corpus callosum
24. Anterior cerebral artery
25. Pericallosal branch of anterior cerebral artery
27. Septum (parolfactory gyrus)
28. Optic nerve
29. Optic chiasm

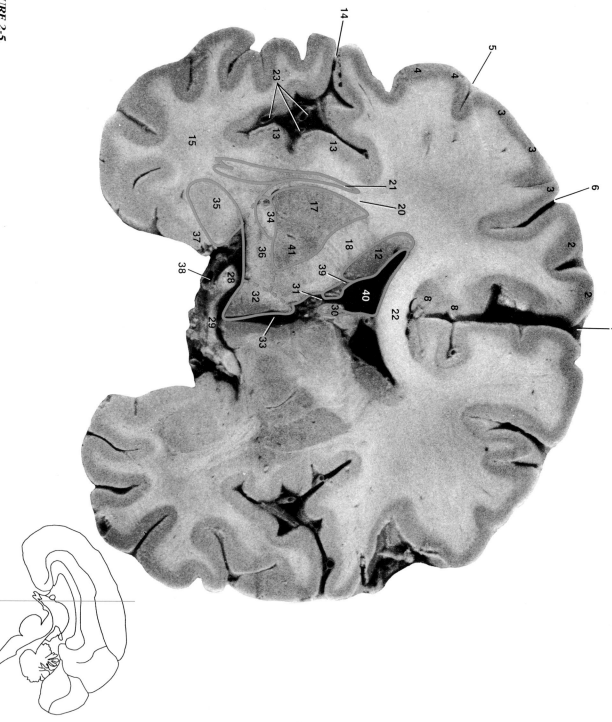

FIGURE 2-5.
Thick coronal section of the brain at the level of the interventricular foramen of Monro.

1. Interhemispheric fissure
2. Superior frontal gyrus
3. Middle frontal gyrus
4. Inferior frontal gyrus
5. Inferior frontal sulcus
6. Superior frontal sulcus
8. Cingulate gyrus
12. Head of caudate nucleus
13. Insula
14. Lateral sulcus (Sylvian fissure)
15. Temporal lobe
17. Putamen
18. Anterior limb of internal capsule
20. External capsule
21. Claustrum
22. Body of corpus callosum
23. Sylvian branches of middle cerebral artery
28. Optic nerve
29. Optic chiasm
30. Fornix
31. Interventricular foramen of Monro
32. Anterior hypothalamus
33. Third ventricle
34. Anterior commissure
35. Amygdala
36. Anterior perforated substance
37. Uncus and parahippocampal gyrus
38. Middle cerebral artery
39. Stria terminalis and thalamostriate (terminal) vein
40. Body of lateral ventricle
41. Globus pallidus

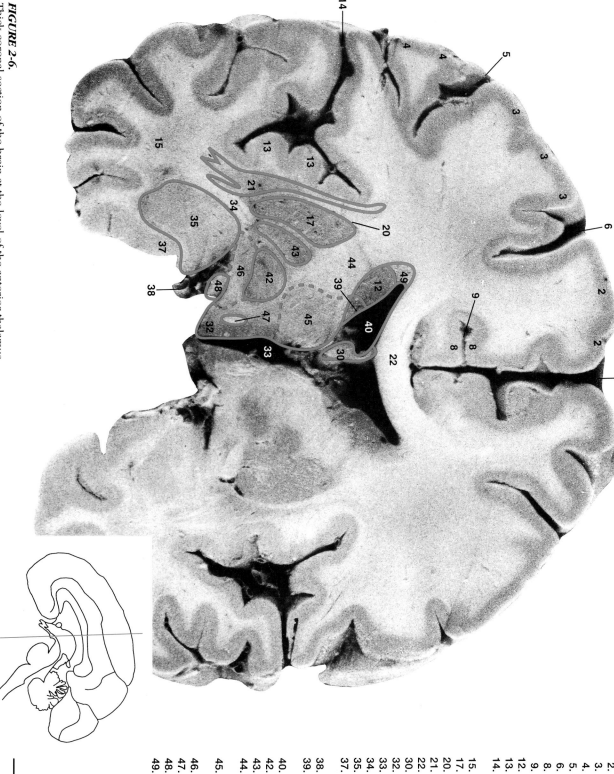

FIGURE 2-6.
Thick coronal section of the brain at the level of the anterior thalamus.

1. Interhemispheric fissure
2. Superior frontal gyrus
3. Middle frontal gyrus
4. Inferior frontal gyrus
5. Inferior frontal sulcus
6. Superior frontal sulcus
8. Cingulate gyrus
9. Cingulate sulcus
12. Head of caudate nucleus
13. Insula
14. Lateral sulcus (Sylvian fissure)
15. Temporal lobe
17. Putamen
20. Claustrum
21. External capsule
22. Body of corpus callosum
30. Fornix
32. Anterior hypothalamus
33. Third ventricle
34. Anterior commissure
35. Amygdala
37. Uncus and parahippocampal gyrus
38. Middle cerebral artery
39. Stria terminalis and thalamostriate (terminal) vein
40. Body of lateral ventricle
42. Globus pallidus I
43. Globus pallidus II
44. Posterior limb of internal capsule
45. Anterior thalamic nuclear group
46. Subthalamus
47. Postcommissural fornix
48. Optic tract
49. Superior longitudinal fasciculus

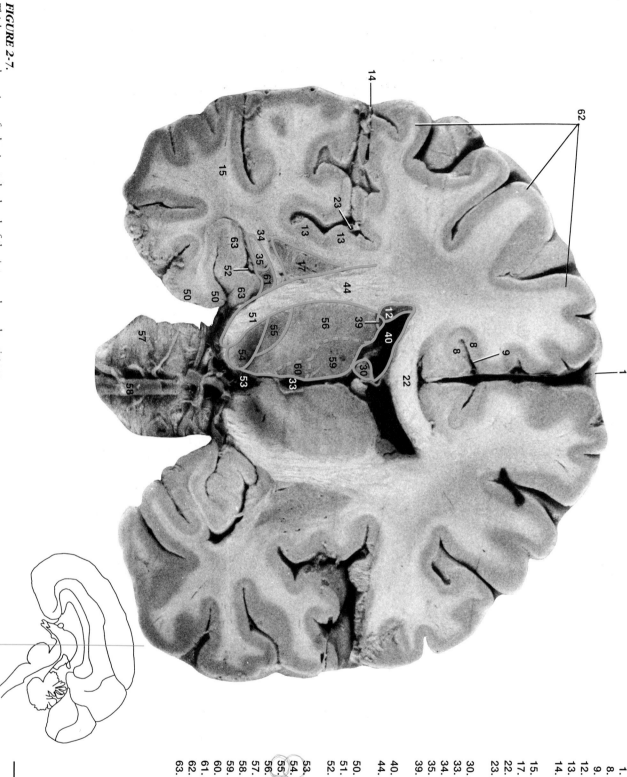

FIGURE 2-7.
Thick coronal section of a brain at the level of the interpeduncular cistern.

1. Interhemispheric fissure
8. Cingulate gyrus
9. Cingulate sulcus
12. Head of caudate nucleus
13. Insula
14. Lateral sulcus (Sylvian fissure)
15. Temporal lobe
17. Putamen
22. Body of corpus callosum
23. Sylvian branches of middle cerebral artery
30. Fornix
33. Third ventricle
34. Anterior commissure
35. Amygdala
39. Stria terminalis and thalamostriate (terminal) vein
40. Body of lateral ventricle
44. Posterior limb of internal capsule
50. Parahippocampal gyrus
51. Cerebral peduncle
52. Inferior horn of lateral ventricle
53. Interpeduncular cistern
54. Substantia nigra
55. Subthalamic nucleus
56. Ventrolateral thalamic nucleus
57. Basilar pons
58. Basilar artery
59. Dorsomedial thalamic nucleus
60. Posterior hypothalamus
61. Lateral geniculate nucleus
62. Parietal lobe
63. Hippocampus

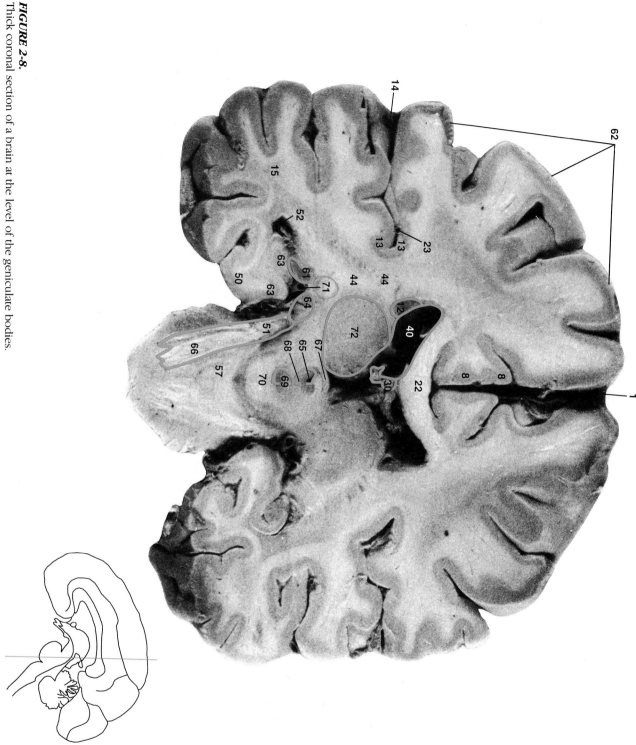

FIGURE 2-8.
Thick coronal section of a brain at the level of the geniculate bodies.

1. Interhemispheric fissure
8. Cingulate gyrus
12. Head of caudate nucleus
13. Insula
14. Lateral sulcus (Sylvian fissure)
15. Temporal lobe
22. Body of corpus callosum
23. Sylvian branches of middle cerebral artery
30. Fornix
40. Body of lateral ventricle
44. Posterior limb of internal capsule
50. Parahippocampal gyrus
51. Cerebral peduncle
52. Inferior horn of lateral ventricle
57. Basilar pons
61. Lateral geniculate nucleus
62. Parietal lobe
63. Hippocampus
64. Medial geniculate nucleus
65. Cerebral aqueduct
66. Pyramidal tract
67. Posterior commissure
68. Periaqueductal gray
69. Interpeduncular nucleus
70. Decussation of superior cerebellar peduncle
71. Posterior cerebral artery
72. Pulvinar

1. Interhemispheric fissure
8. Cingulate gyrus
9. Cingulate sulcus
73. Trigone of lateral ventricle
74. Middle cerebellar peduncle
75. Superior cerebellum
76. Inferior cerebellum
77. Choroid plexus in trigone
78. Superior cerebellar peduncle
79. Pons
80. Medulla
81. Fourth ventricle
82. Quadrigeminal cistern
83. Internal cerebral vein
84. Geniculo-calcarine tract
    (visual pathway)
85. Splenium of corpus callosum

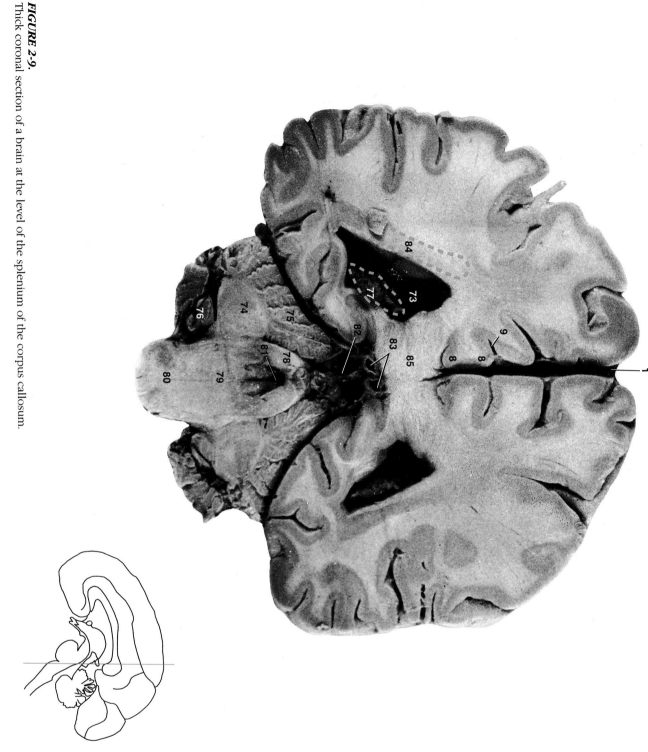

FIGURE 2-9.
Thick coronal section of a brain at the level of the splenium of the corpus callosum.

Coronal Sections of the Brain
(Myelin Stain)

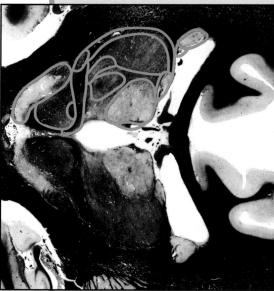

Atlas of the Human Brain, by Lothar Jennes, Harold H. Traurig, and P. Michael Conn. J. B. Lippincott Company, Philadelphia, © 1995.

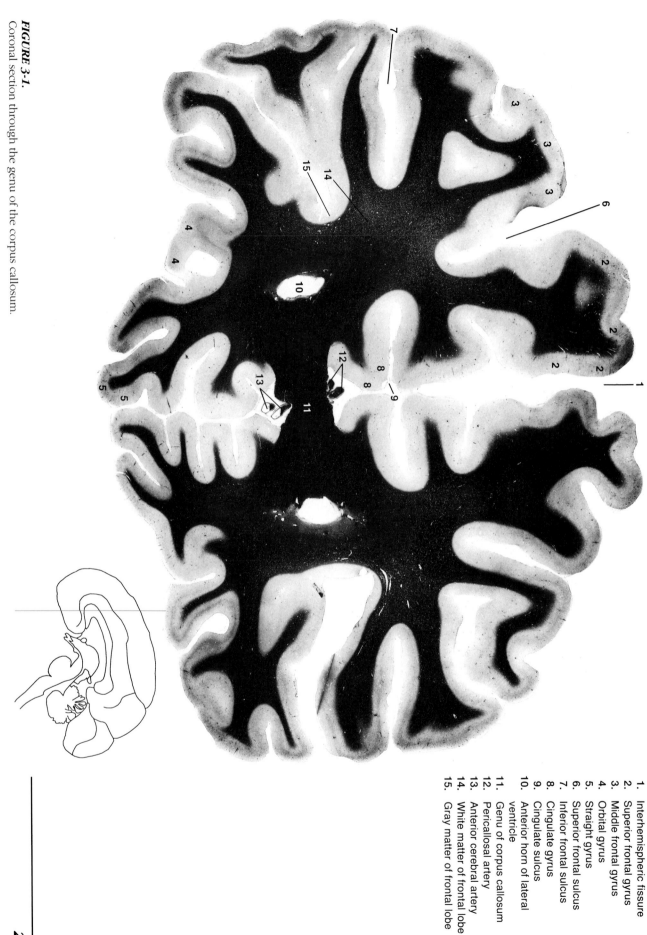

FIGURE 3-1.
Coronal section through the genu of the corpus callosum.

1. Interhemispheric fissure
2. Superior frontal gyrus
3. Middle frontal gyrus
4. Orbital gyrus
5. Straight gyrus
6. Superior frontal sulcus
7. Inferior frontal sulcus
8. Cingulate gyrus
9. Cingulate sulcus
10. Anterior horn of lateral ventricle
11. Genu of corpus callosum
12. Pericallosal artery
13. Anterior cerebral artery
14. White matter of frontal lobe
15. Gray matter of frontal lobe

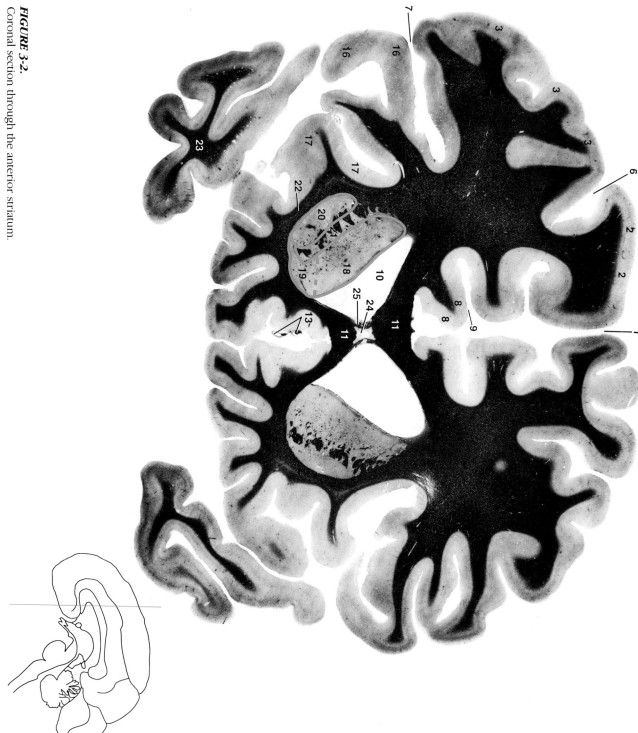

FIGURE 3-2.
Coronal section through the anterior striatum.

1. Interhemispheric fissure
2. Superior frontal gyrus
3. Middle frontal gyrus
6. Superior frontal sulcus
7. Inferior frontal sulcus
8. Cingulate gyrus
9. Cingulate sulcus
10. Anterior horn of lateral ventricle
11. Genu of corpus callosum
13. Anterior cerebral artery
16. Inferior frontal gyrus
17. Insula
18. Head of caudate nucleus
19. Nucleus accumbens
20. Putamen
21. Anterior limb of internal capsule
22. External capsule
23. Temporal lobe
24. Cavum of septum pellucidum
25. Septum pellucidum

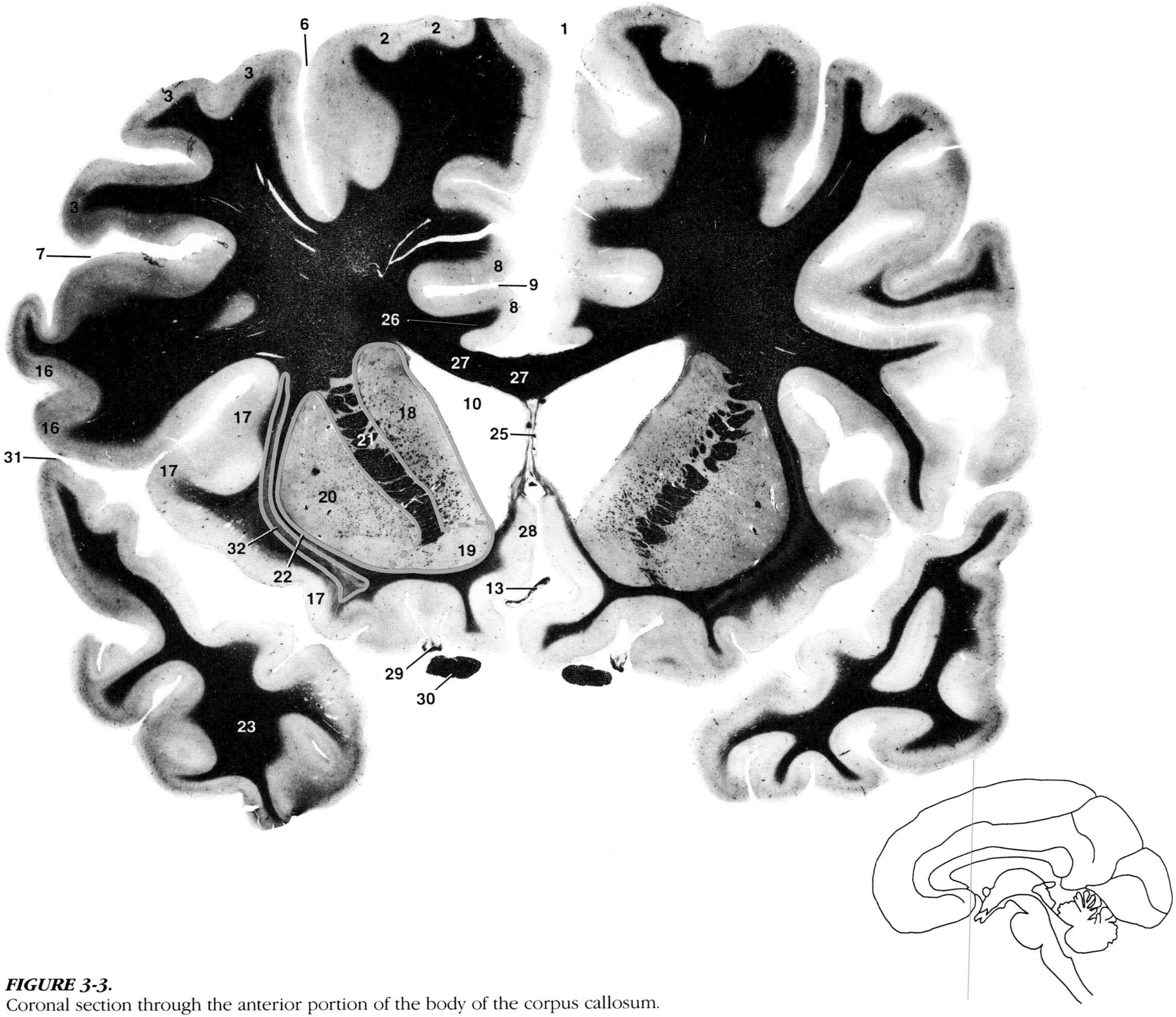

FIGURE 3-3.
Coronal section through the anterior portion of the body of the corpus callosum.

1. Interhemispheric fissure
2. Superior frontal gyrus
3. Middle frontal gyrus
6. Superior frontal sulcus
7. Inferior frontal sulcus
8. Cingulate gyrus
9. Cingulate sulcus
10. Anterior horn of lateral
    ventricle
13. Anterior cerebral artery
16. Inferior frontal gyrus
17. Insula
18. Head of caudate nucleus
19. Putamen
20. Nucleus accumbens
21. Anterior limb of internal
    capsule
22. External capsule
23. Temporal lobe
25. Septum pellucidum
26. Cingulum
27. Body of corpus callosum
28. Septum (parolfactory gyrus)
29. Olfactory tract
30. Optic nerve (II)
31. Lateral sulcus (Sylvian
    fissure)
32. Claustrum

1. Interhemispheric fissure
8. Cingulate gyrus
9. Cingulate sulcus
10. Anterior horn of lateral ventricle
17. Insula
18. Head of caudate nucleus
20. Putamen
21. Anterior limb of internal capsule
22. External capsule
26. Cingulum
27. Body of corpus callosum
31. Lateral sulcus (Sylvian fissure)
32. Claustrum
33. Globus pallidus
34. Fornix
35. Anterior commissure
36. Stria terminalis
37. Bed nucleus of stria terminalis
38. Preoptic nuclei
39. Optic chiasm
40. Third ventricle
41. Infundibular stalk
42. Internal carotid artery (branchpoint: anterior and middle cerebral arteries)
43. Amygdala complex
44. Olfactory tubercle (anterior perforated substance)
45. Uncus

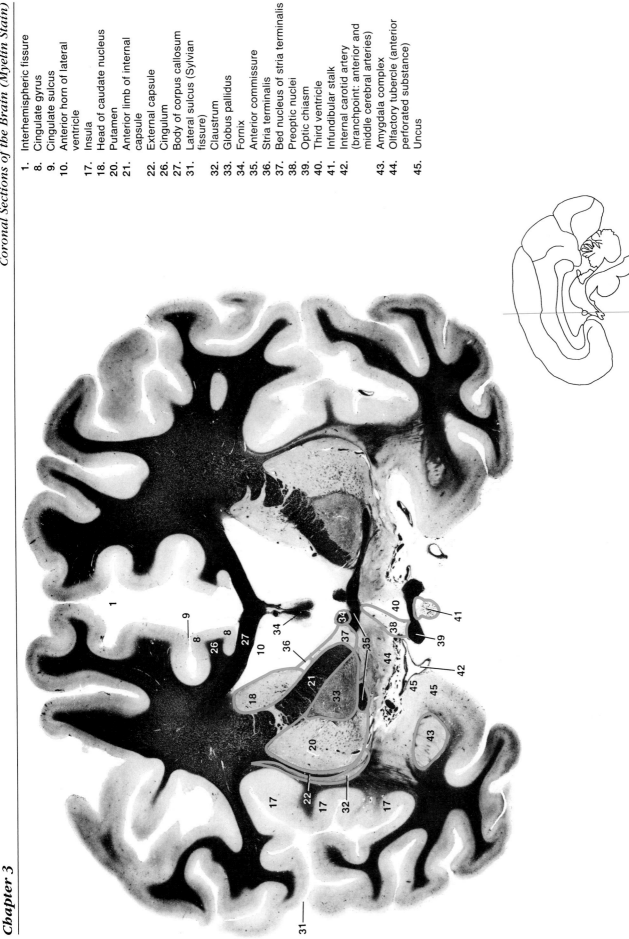

FIGURE 3-4.
Coronal section through the optic chiasm and anterior commissure.

Coronal Sections of the Brain (Myelin Stain)

1. Interhemispheric fissure
8. Cingulate gyrus
9. Cingulate sulcus
17. Insula
20. Putamen
22. External capsule
26. Cingulum
27. Body of corpus callosum
31. Lateral sulcus (Sylvian fissure)
32. Claustrum
34. Fornix
35. Anterior commissure
36. Stria terminalis
40. Third ventricle
43. Amygdala complex
45. Uncus
46. Body of caudate nucleus
47. Interventricular foramen of Monro
48. Globus pallidus I
49. Globus pallidus II
50. Posterior limb of internal capsule
51. Ansa lenticularis
52. Optic tract
53. Hypothalamus
54. Anterior nuclei of thalamus
55. Stria medullaris of thalamus
56. Inferior horn of lateral ventricle
57. Body of lateral ventricle

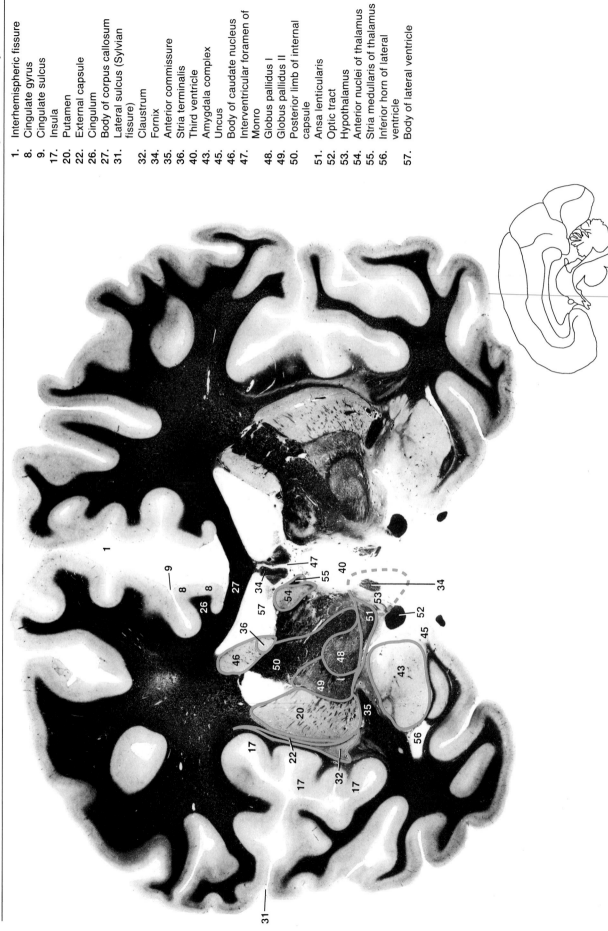

FIGURE 3-5.

Coronal section through the interventricular foramen of Monro.

1. Interhemispheric fissure
8. Cingulate gyrus
9. Cingulate sulcus
17. Insula
20. Putamen
22. External capsule
26. Cingulum
27. Body of corpus callosum
31. Lateral sulcus (Sylvian fissure)
32. Claustrum
34. Fornix
36. Stria terminalis
43. Amygdala complex
46. Body of caudate nucleus
48. Globus pallidus I
49. Globus pallidus II
50. Posterior limb of internal capsule
52. Optic tract
54. Anterior nuclei of thalamus
55. Stria medullaris of thalamus
56. Inferior horn of lateral ventricle
57. Body of lateral ventricle
58. Oculomotor nerve (III)
59. Internal cerebral vein
60. Ventral lateral nucleus of thalamus
61. Mammillo-thalamic tract
62. Dorsomedial nucleus of thalamus
63. Midline nuclear group of thalamus
64. Internal medullary lamina
65. Subthalamus
66. Lenticular fasciculus, H2 field of Forel
67. Posterior hypothalamus
68. Cerebral peduncle
69. Medial forebrain bundle
70. Mammillary body
71. Parahippocampal gyrus
72. Pes hippocampi

31

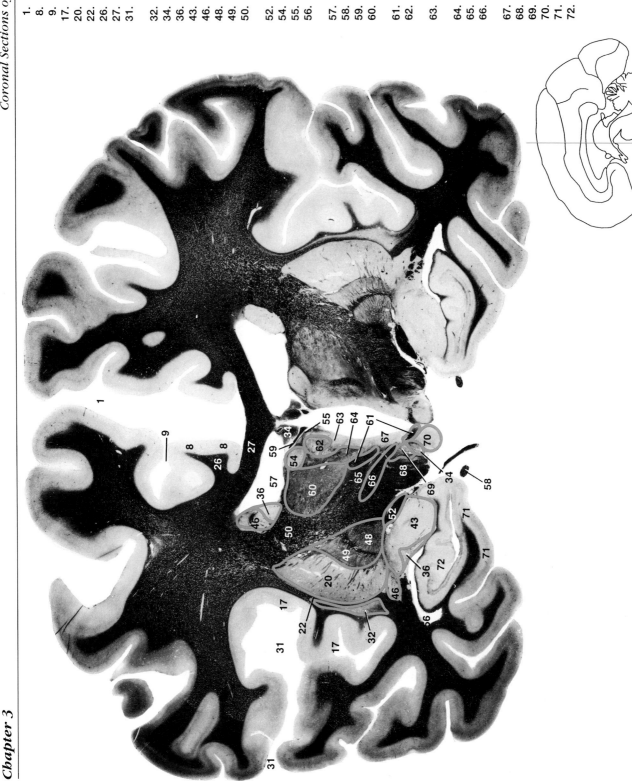

FIGURE 3-6.
Coronal section through the anterior thalamus.

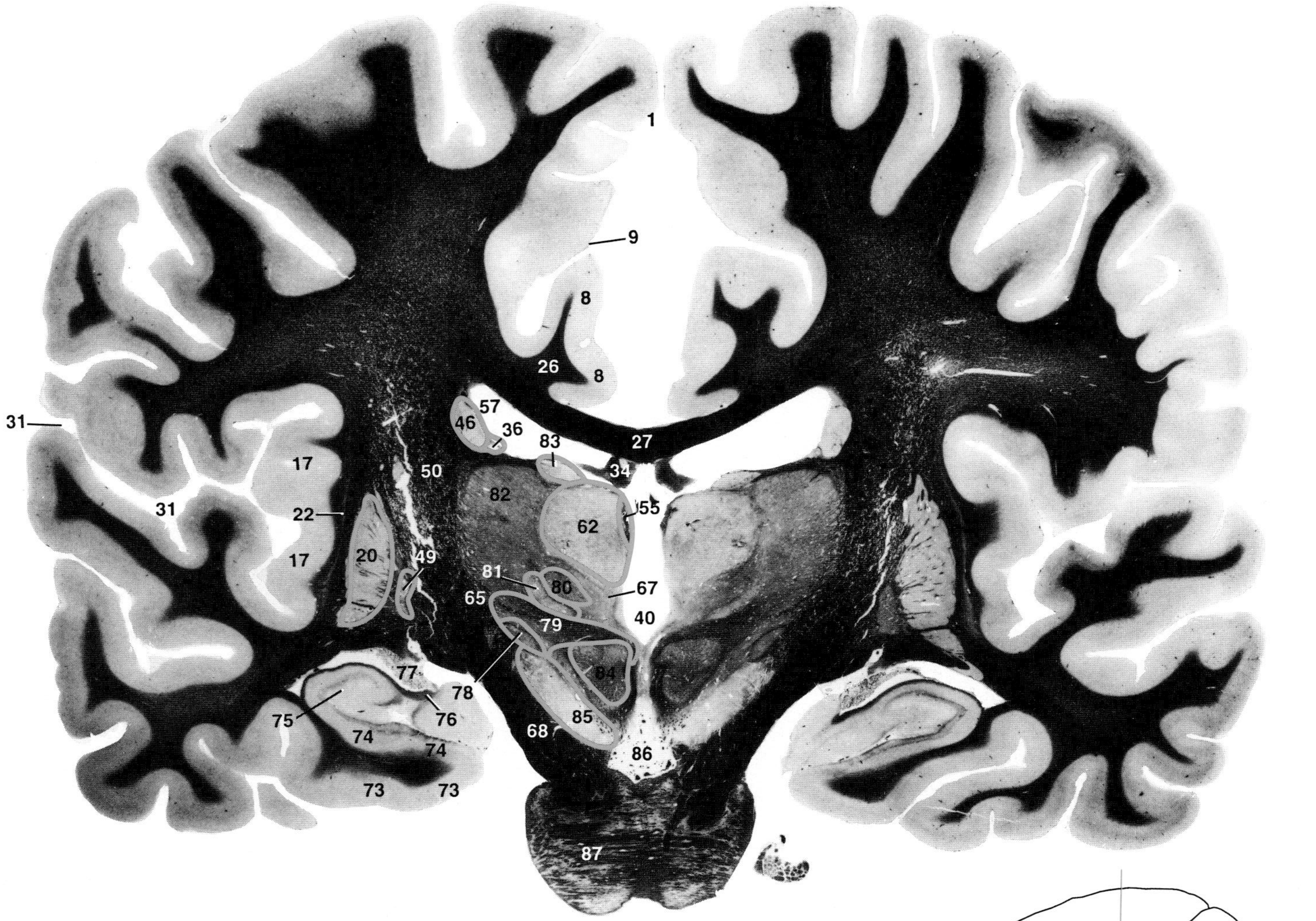

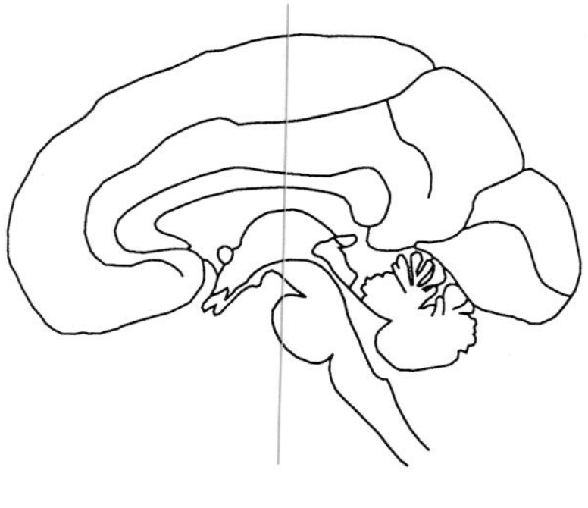

1. Interhemispheric fissure
8. Cingulate gyrus
9. Cingulate sulcus
17. Insula
20. Putamen
22. External capsule
26. Cingulum
27. Body of corpus callosum
31. Lateral sulcus (Sylvian fissure)
34. Fornix
36. Stria terminalis
40. Third ventricle
46. Body of caudate nucleus
49. Globus pallidus II
50. Posterior limb of internal capsule
55. Stria medullaris of thalamus
57. Body of lateral ventricle
62. Dorsomedial nucleus of thalamus
65. Subthalamus
67. Posterior hypothalamus
68. Cerebral peduncle
73. Entorhinal cortex
74. Subiculum
75. Hippocampus
76. Fimbria of fornix
77. Choroid plexus in inferior horn of lateral ventricle
78. Subthalamic nucleus
79. Dentato-rubro-thalamic track and thalamic fasciculus (H1)
80. Centro-median nucleus of thalamus
81. Ventral posterior nucleus of thalamus
82. Lateral posterior nucleus of thalamus
83. Lateral dorsal nucleus of thalamus
84. Red nucleus
85. Substantia nigra
86. Interpeduncular cistern
87. Basilar pons

32

FIGURE 3-7.
Coronal section through the mid-thalamus.

Coronal Sections of the Brain (Myelin Stain)

1. Interhemispheric fissure
8. Cingulate gyrus
9. Cingulate sulcus
17. Insula
20. Putamen
22. External capsule
26. Cingulum
27. Body of corpus callosum
31. Lateral sulcus (Sylvian fissure)
34. Fornix
36. Stria terminalis
40. Third ventricle
46. Body of caudate nucleus
50. Posterior limb of internal capsule
55. Stria medullaris of thalamus
57. Body of lateral ventricle
62. Dorsomedial nucleus of thalamus
65. Subthalamus
67. Posterior hypothalamus
68. Cerebral peduncle
73. Entorhinal cortex
74. Subiculum
75. Hippocampus
76. Fimbria of fornix
77. Choroid plexus in inferior horn of lateral ventricle
78. Subthalamic nucleus
79. Dentato-rubro-thalamic track and thalamic fasciculus (H1)
80. Centro-median nucleus of thalamus
81. Ventral posterior nucleus of thalamus
82. Lateral posterior nucleus of thalamus
83. Lateral dorsal nucleus of thalamus
84. Red nucleus
85. Substantia nigra
86. Interpeduncular cistern
87. Basilar pons
88. Fasciculus retroflexus
89. Internal medullary lamina
90. External medullary lamina and thalamic reticular nuclei
91. Tail of caudate nucleus.

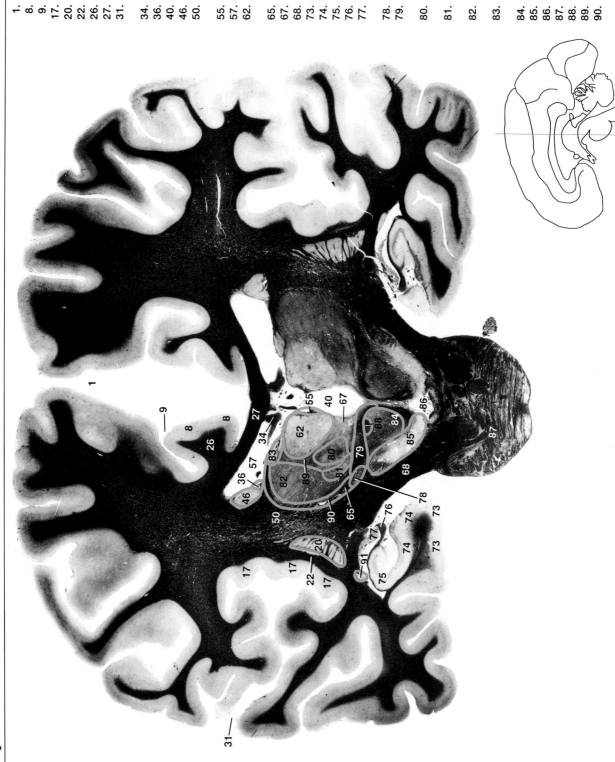

FIGURE 3-8.
Coronal section through the posterior thalamus.

33

Coronal Sections of the Brain (Myelin Stain)

1. Interhemispheric fissure
8. Cingulate gyrus
9. Cingulate sulcus
17. Insula
20. Putamen
22. External capsule
26. Cingulum
27. Body of corpus callosum
31. Lateral sulcus (Sylvian fissure)
34. Fornix
36. Stria terminalis
40. Third ventricle
46. Body of caudate nucleus
50. Posterior limb of internal capsule
57. Body of lateral ventricle
62. Dorsomedial nucleus of thalamus
67. Posterior hypothalamus
68. Cerebral peduncle
73. Entorhinal cortex
74. Subiculum
75. Hippocampus
76. Fimbria of fornix
77. Choroid plexus in inferior horn of lateral ventricle
79. Dentato-rubro-thalamic track and thalamic fasciculus (H1)
80. Centro-median nucleus of thalamus
81. Ventral posterior nucleus of thalamus
82. Lateral posterior nucleus of thalamus
83. Lateral dorsal nucleus of thalamus
84. Red nucleus
85. Substantia nigra
86. Interpeduncular cistern
87. Basilar pons
89. Internal medullary lamina
90. External medullary lamina and thalamic reticular nuclei
91. Tail of caudate nucleus
92. Zona incerta
93. Habenula
94. Lateral geniculate nucleus

34

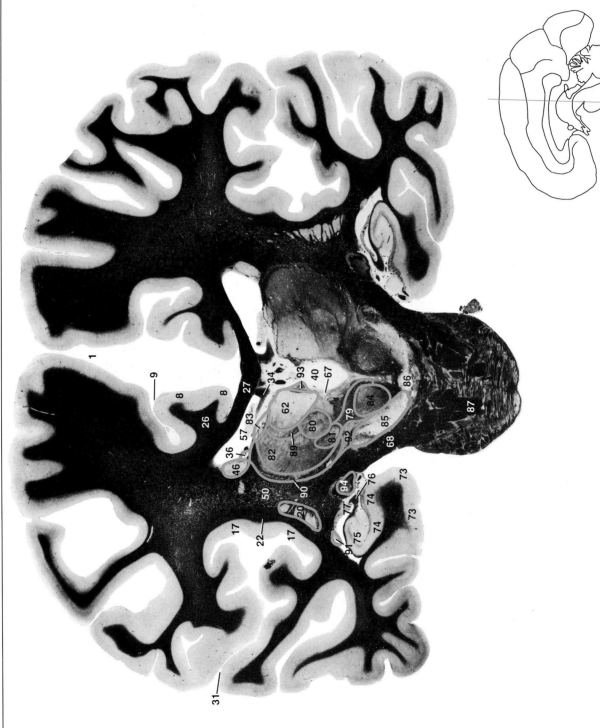

FIGURE 3-9.
Coronal section through the posterior thalamus and habenula.

1. Interhemispheric fissure
8. Cingulate gyrus
9. Cingulate sulcus
17. Insula
22. External capsule
26. Cingulum
27. Body of corpus callosum
31. Lateral sulcus (Sylvian fissure)
34. Fornix
36. Stria terminalis
46. Body of caudate nucleus
50. Posterior limb of internal capsule
57. Body of lateral ventricle
62. Dorsomedial nucleus of thalamus
68. Cerebral peduncle
73. Entorhinal cortex
74. Subiculum
75. Hippocampus
76. Fimbria of fornix
83. Lateral dorsal nucleus of thalamus
87. Basilar pons
90. External medullary lamina and thalamic reticular nuclei
94. Lateral geniculate nucleus
95. Pulvinar
96. Pineal
97. Habenular commissure
98. Posterior commissure
99. Cerebral aqueduct
100. Periaqueductal gray
101. Oculomotor nucleus (III)
102. Decussation of superior cerebellar peduncle
103. Pontocerebellar tract
104. Middle cerebellar peduncle
105. Roots of trigeminal nerve (V)
106. Pyramidal tract
107. Medial lemniscus
108. Spinothalamic tract
109. Lateral lemniscus
110. Medial geniculate nucleus
111. Posterior thalamic radiations (geniculo-calcarine tract)

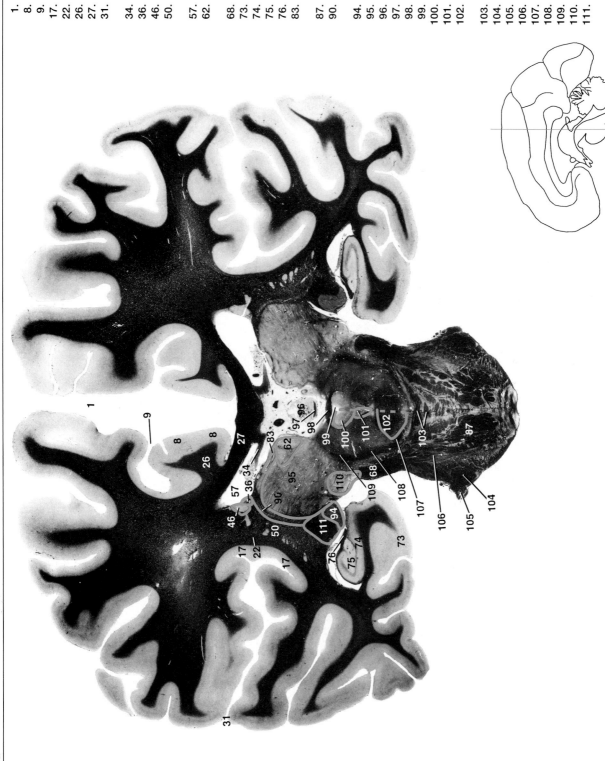

FIGURE 3-10.
Coronal section through the pulvinar and geniculi.

Coronal Sections of the Brain (Myelin Stain)

1. Interhemispheric fissure
8. Cingulate gyrus
9. Cingulate sulcus
17. Insula
26. Cingulum
27. Body of corpus callosum
31. Lateral sulcus (Sylvian fissure)
34. Fornix
46. Body of caudate nucleus
57. Body of lateral ventricle
74. Subiculum
75. Hippocampus
76. Fimbria of fornix
87. Basilar pons
90. External medullary lamina and thalamic reticular nuclei
95. Pulvinar
99. Cerebral aqueduct
100. Periaqueductal gray
103. Pontocerebellar tract
104. Middle cerebellar peduncle
106. Pyramidal tract
112. Quadrigeminal cistern
113. Superior colliculus
114. Medial longitudinal fascicle
115. Pontine reticular formation
116. Pontine nuclei
117. Cerebellar hemisphere

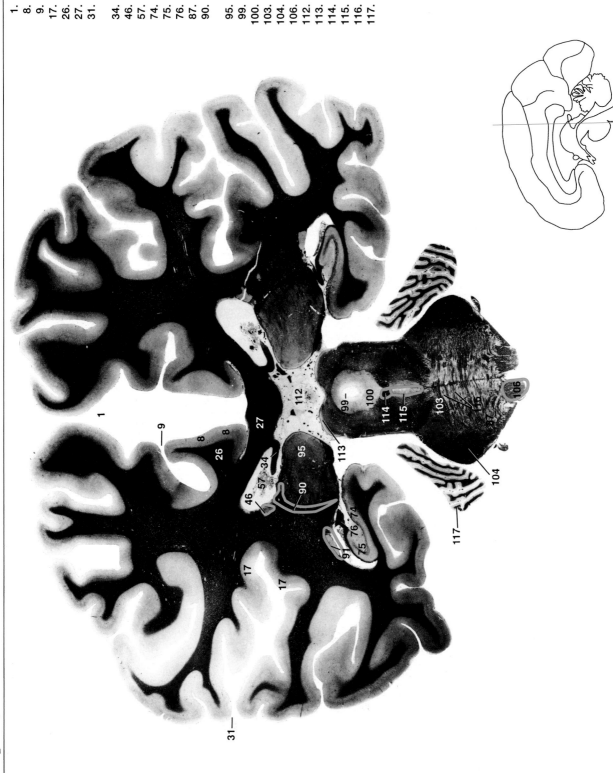

FIGURE 3-11.
Coronal section through the pulvinar and most posterior extent of the body of the lateral ventricle.

Coronal Sections of the Brain (Myelin Stain)

1. Interhemispheric fissure
8. Cingulate gyrus
26. Cingulum
46. Body of caudate nucleus
75. Hippocampus
76. Fimbria of fornix
99. Cerebral aqueduct
100. Periaqueductal gray
104. Middle cerebellar peduncle
106. Pyramidal tract
112. Quadrigeminal cistern
113. Superior colliculus
114. Medial longitudinal fascicle
117. Cerebellar hemisphere
118. Commissure of superior colliculus
119. Pontine reticular formation, central nucleus, and nucleus gigantocellularis
120. Inferior olivary nucleus
121. Facial nucleus
122. Roots of facial nerve (VII)
123. Motor nucleus of trigeminal nerve (V)
124. Central tegmental tract
125. Superior cerebellar peduncle
126. Splenium of corpus callosum
127. Trigone of lateral ventricle

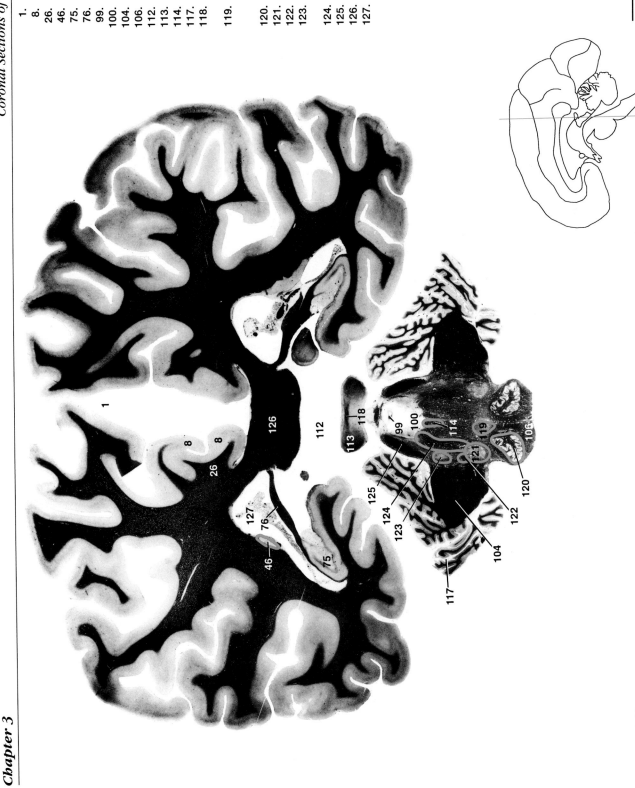

FIGURE 3-12.
Coronal section through the splenium of the corpus callosum and the confluence of lateral ventricles.

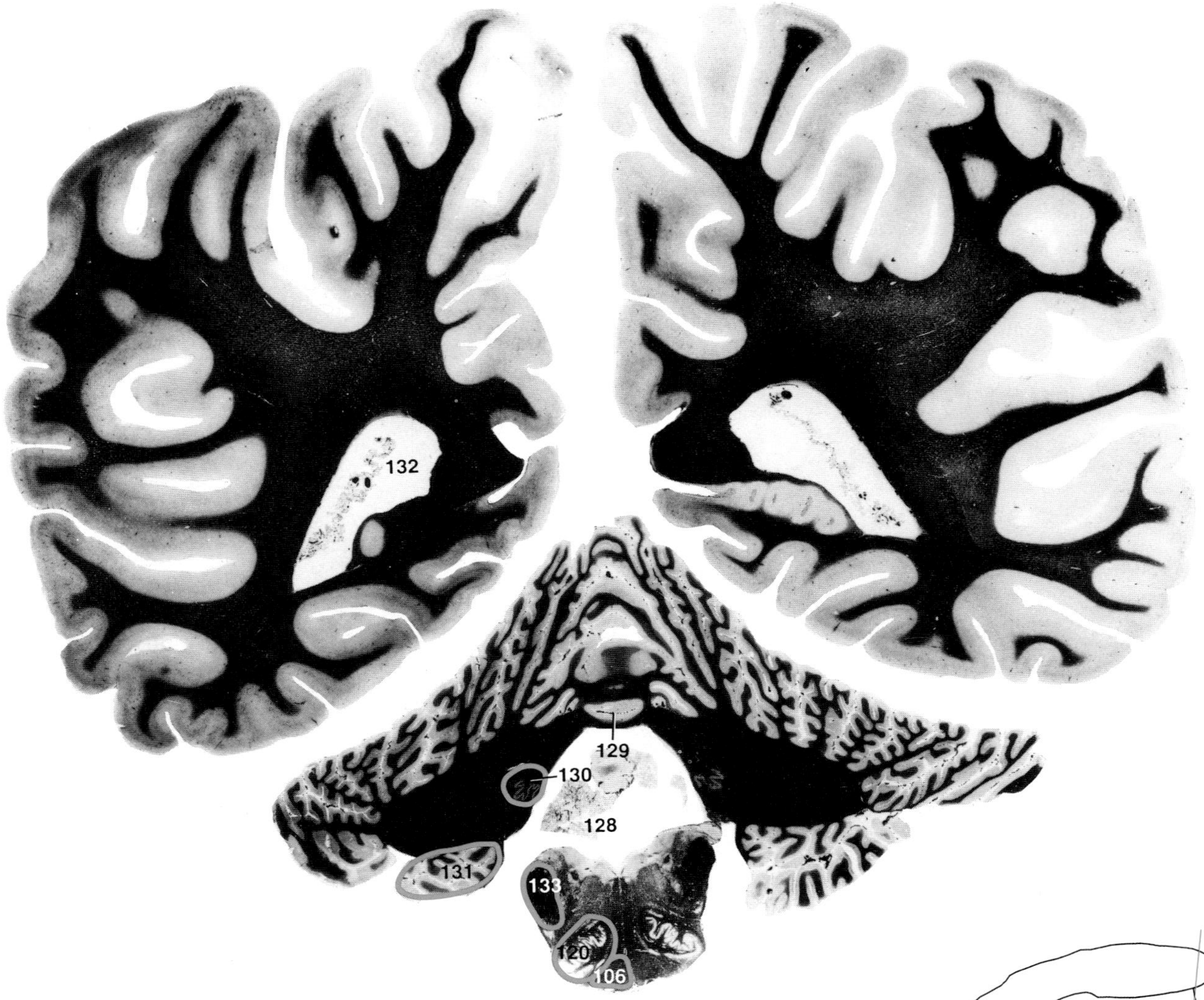

Coronal Sections of the Brain (Myelin Stain)

106. Pyramidal tract
120. Inferior olivary nucleus
128. Fourth ventricle
129. Vermis of cerebellum
130. Dentate nucleus
131. Tonsil of cerebellum
132. Posterior horn of lateral ventricle
133. Inferior cerebellar peduncle

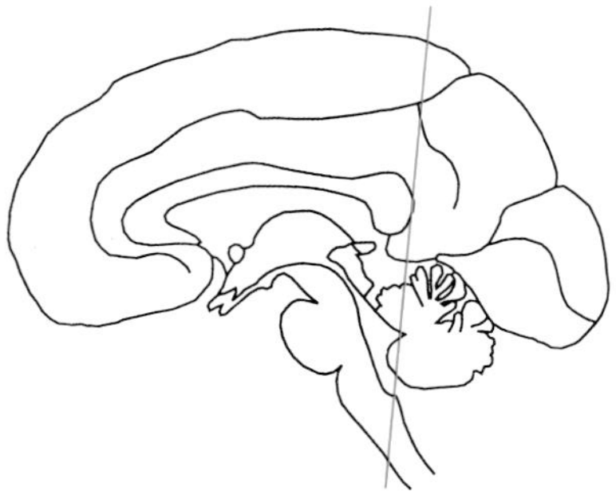

FIGURE 3-13.
Coronal section through the parietal lobe posterior to the splenium.

Coronal Sections of the Brain (Myelin Stain)

106. Pyramidal tract
128. Fourth ventricle
129. Vermis of cerebellum
130. Dentate nucleus
131. Tonsil of cerebellum
132. Posterior horn of lateral ventricle
134. Globose nucleus
135. Emboliform nucleus
136. Fastigial nucleus
137. Optic radiations

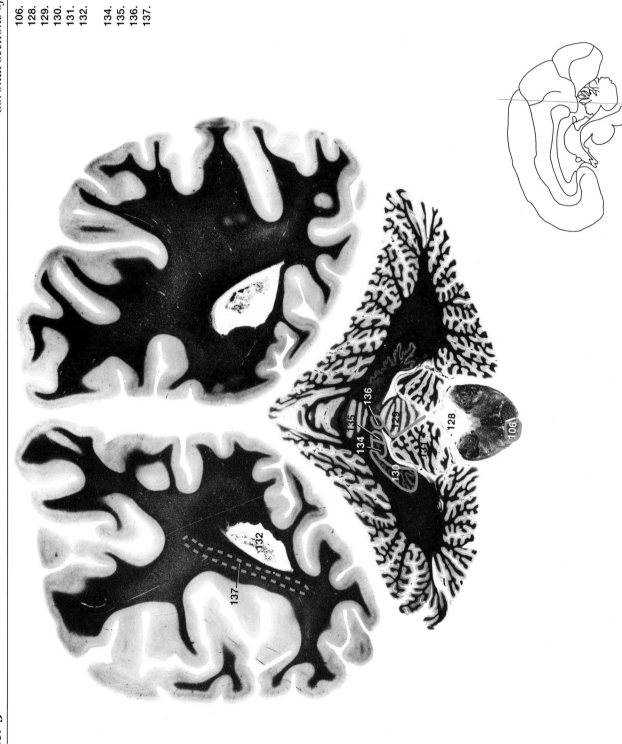

FIGURE 3-14.
Coronal section through the occipital lobe and posterior horn of the lateral ventricle.

39

138. Visual (calcarine) cortex,
     band of Gennari
139. C1 spinal cord

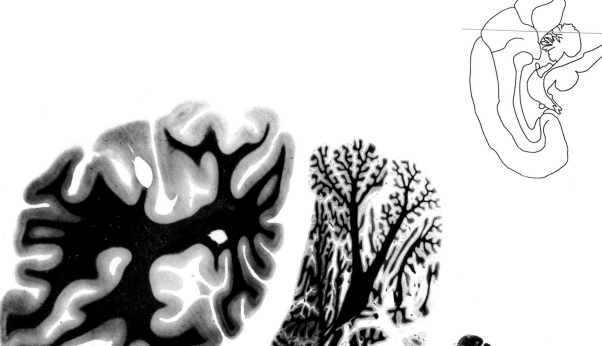

138

139

FIGURE 3-15.
Coronal section through the occipital lobe posterior to the posterior horn of the lateral ventricle.

Atlas of the Human Brain, by Lothar Jennes,
Harold H. Traurig, and P. Michael Conn.
J. B. Lippincott Company, Philadelphia. © 1995.

Horizontal Sections of the Brain (Myelin Stain)

c h a p t e r **4**

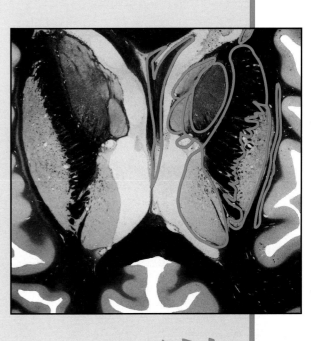

Horizontal Sections of the Brain (Myelin Stain)

1. Frontal pole
2. Occipital pole
3. Interhemispheric fissure
4. Cingulate gyrus
5. Genu of corpus callosum
6. Anterior horn of lateral ventricle
7. Body of lateral ventricle
8. Body of corpus callosum
9. Stria terminalis
10. Head of caudate nucleus
11. Body of caudate nucleus
12. Insula
13. Anterior limb of internal capsule
14. Splenium of corpus callosum
15. Visual (calcarine) cortex, band of Gennari

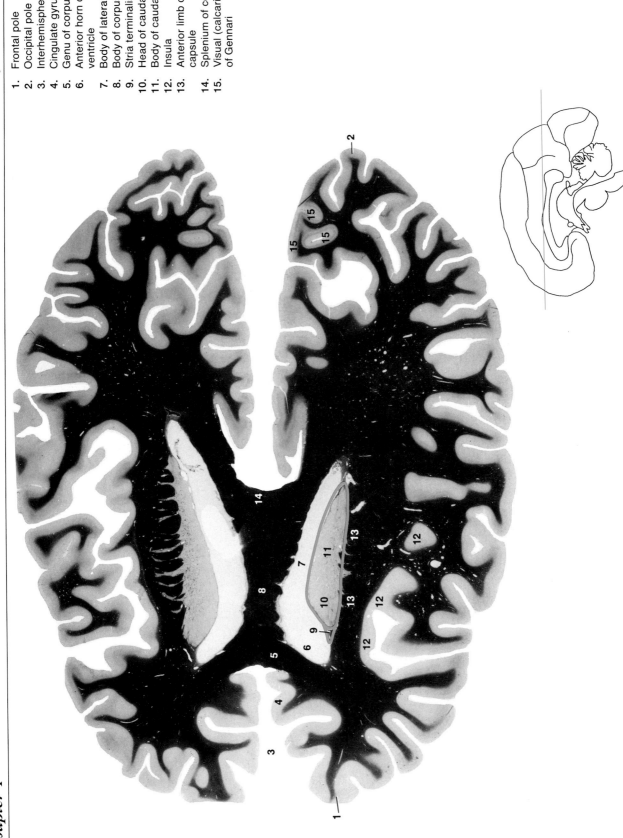

FIGURE 4-1.
Horizontal section through the body of the corpus callosum.

Horizontal Sections of the Brain (Myelin Stain)

1. Frontal pole
2. Occipital pole
3. Interhemispheric fissure
4. Cingulate gyrus
5. Genu of corpus callosum
6. Anterior horn of lateral ventricle
7. Body of lateral ventricle
9. Stria terminalis
10. Head of caudate nucleus
12. Insula
13. Anterior limb of internal capsule
14. Splenium of corpus callosum
15. Visual (calcarine) cortex, band of Gennari
16. Putamen
17. Genu of internal capsule
18. Posterior limb of internal capsule
19. External medullary lamina and thalamic reticular nuclei
20. Lateral thalamic nucleus
21. Internal medullary lamina
22. Anterior thalamic nucleus
23. Thalamostriatal vein
24. External capsule
25. Claustrum
26. Septum pellucidum
27. Septum (parolfactory gyrus)
28. Crus of fornix
29. Lateral dorsal thalamic nucleus
30. Tail of caudate nucleus
31. Posterior horn of lateral ventricle

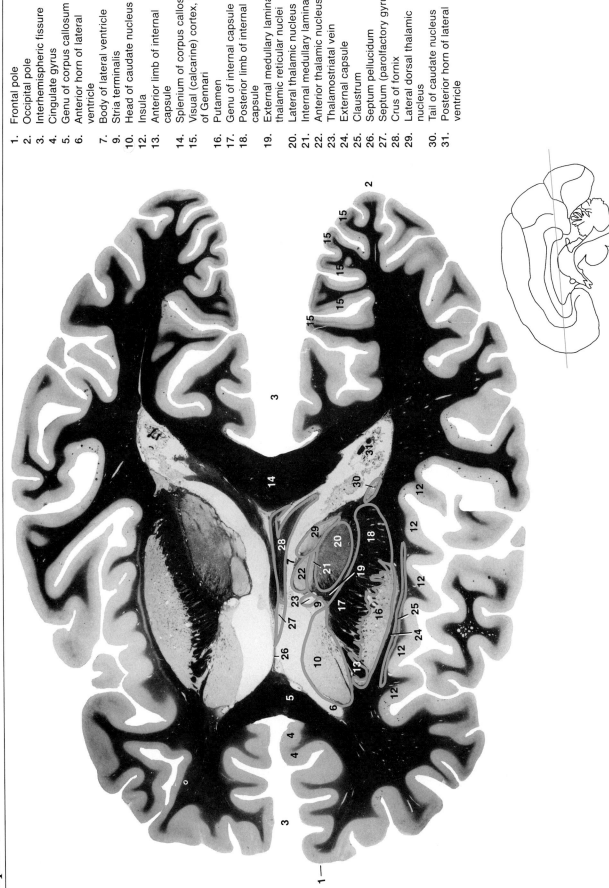

FIGURE 4-2.
Horizontal section through the superior thalamus.

1. Frontal pole
2. Occipital pole
3. Interhemispheric fissure
4. Cingulate gyrus
5. Genu of corpus callosum
6. Anterior horn of lateral ventricle
9. Stria terminalis
10. Head of caudate nucleus
12. Insula
13. Anterior limb of internal capsule
14. Splenium of corpus callosum
15. Visual (calcarine) cortex, band of Gennari
16. Putamen
17. Genu of internal capsule
18. Posterior limb of internal capsule
19. External medullary lamina and thalamic reticular nuclei
21. Internal medullary lamina
22. Anterior thalamic nucleus
24. External capsule
25. Claustrum
27. Septum (parolfactory gyrus)
28. Crus of fornix
30. Tail of caudate nucleus
31. Posterior horn of lateral ventricle
32. Body of fornix
33. Interventricular foramen of Monro
34. Third ventricle
35. Ventral anterior thalamic nucleus
36. Ventral lateral thalamic nucleus
37. Lateral posterior thalamic nucleus
38. Pulvinar
39. Dorsal medial thalamic nucleus

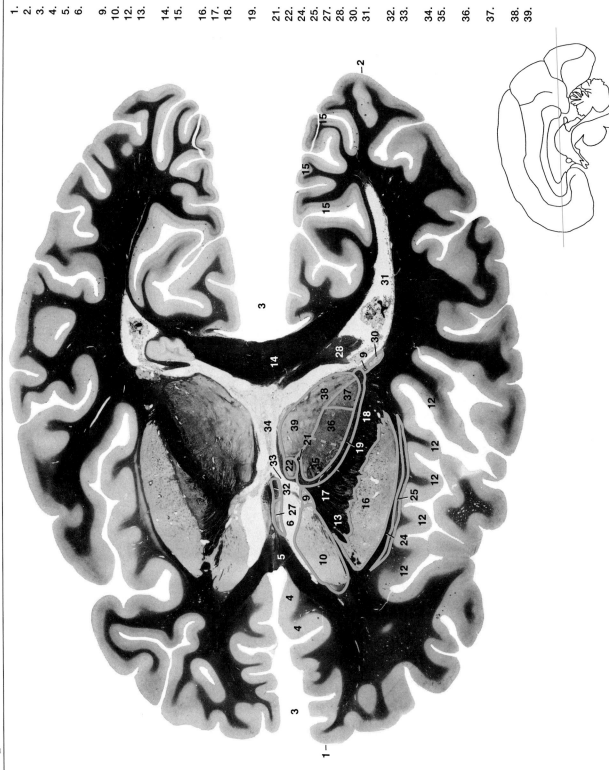

FIGURE 4-3.

Horizontal section through the interventricular foramen of Monro.

Horizontal Sections of the Brain (Myelin Stain)

1. Frontal pole
2. Occipital pole
3. Interhemispheric fissure
9. Stria terminalis
10. Head of caudate nucleus
12. Insula
13. Anterior limb of internal capsule
15. Visual (calcarine) cortex, band of Gennari
16. Putamen
18. Posterior limb of internal capsule
24. External capsule
25. Claustrum
30. Tail of caudate nucleus
34. Third ventricle
36. Ventral lateral thalamic nucleus
37. Lateral posterior thalamic nucleus
38. Pulvinar
39. Dorsal medial thalamic nucleus
40. Paraterminal gyrus
41. Parolfactory cortex
42. Anterior commissure
43. Column of fornix
44. Hypothalamus
45. Massa intermedia
46. Lateral medullary lamina of globus pallidus
47. Medial medullary lamina of globus pallidus
48. Globus pallidus II
49. Globus pallidus I
50. Mammillothalamic tract
51. Ansa lenticularis
52. Centromedian thalamic nucleus
53. Optic radiations
54. Habenula
55. Habenular commissure
56. Pineal
57. Quadrigeminal cistern
58. Fimbria of fornix
59. Hippocampus
60. Trigone of lateral ventricle

45

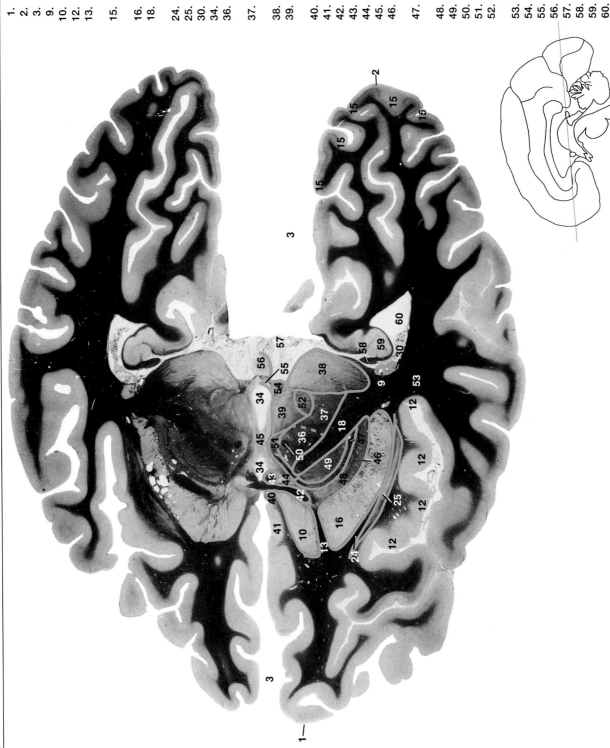

FIGURE 4-4.
Horizontal section through the anterior commissure and pineal.

Horizontal Sections of the Brain (Myelin Stain)

1. Frontal pole
2. Occipital pole
3. Interhemispheric fissure
12. Insula
30. Tail of caudate nucleus
34. Third ventricle
43. Column of fornix
44. Hypothalamus
50. Mammillothalamic tract
51. Ansa lenticularis
53. Optic radiations
58. Fimbria of fornix
59. Hippocampus
61. Anterior cerebral artery
62. Lamina terminalis
63. Amygdala
64. Optic tract
65. Cerebral peduncle
66. Subthalamic nucleus
67. Dentato-rubro-thalamic tract
68. Red nucleus
69. Fasciculus retroflexus
70. Medial leminiscus
71. Lateral geniculate nucleus
72. Medial geniculate nucleus
73. Periaqueductal gray
74. Cerebral aqueduct
75. Superior colliculus
76. Parahippocampal gyrus
77. Inferior horn of lateral ventricle
78. Vermis of cerebellum

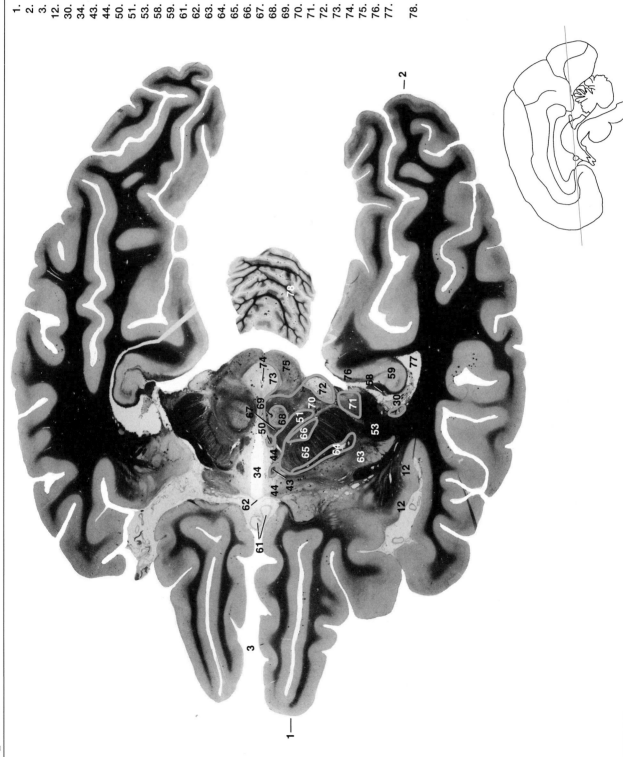

FIGURE 4-5.
Horizontal section through the base of the cerebrum, hypothalamus, and midbrain.

Horizontal Sections of the Brain (Myelin Stain)

2. Occipital pole
3. Interhemispheric fissure
9. Stria terminalis
30. Tail of caudate nucleus
34. Third ventricle
43. Column of fornix
44. Hypothalamus
50. Mammillo-thalamic tract
58. Fimbria of fornix
59. Hippocampus
61. Anterior cerebral artery
62. Lamina terminalis
63. Amygdala
64. Optic tract
65. Cerebral peduncle
66. Subthalamic nucleus
67. Dentato-rubro-thalamic tract
68. Red nucleus
69. Fasciculus retroflexus
70. Medial lemniscus
71. Lateral geniculate nucleus
72. Medial geniculate nucleus
73. Periaqueductal gray
74. Cerebral aqueduct
75. Superior colliculus
76. Parahippocampal gyrus
77. Inferior horn of lateral
    ventricle
78. Vermis of cerebellum
79. Substantia nigra
80. Spinothalamic tract
81. Brachium of inferior colliculus
82. Reticular formation
83. Decussation of superior
    colliculus
84. Oculomotor nucleus (III)

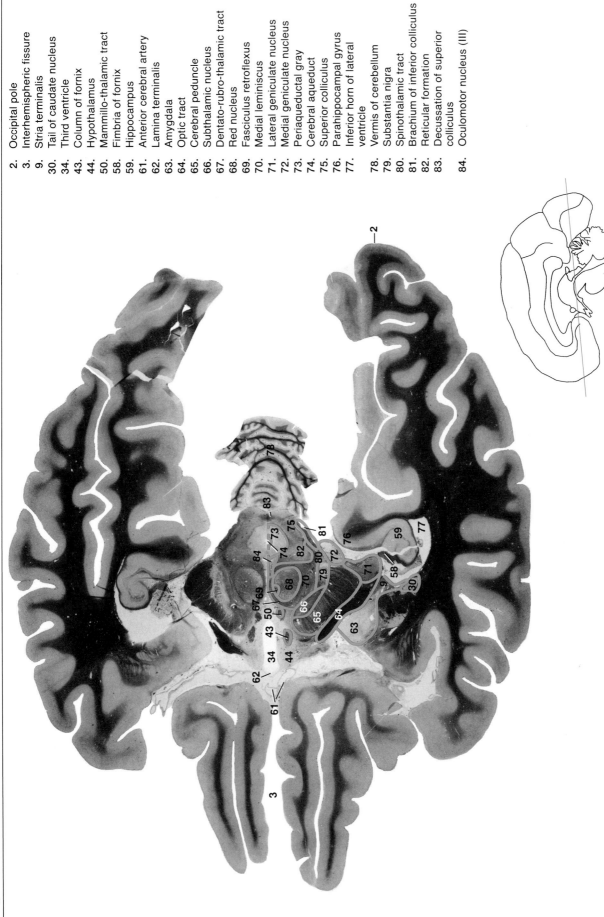

FIGURE 4-6.

Horizontal section through the base of the cerebrum, hypothalamus and midbrain at the level of the decussation of the superior colliculus, just inferior to section shown in Figure 4-5.

Horizontal Sections of the Brain (Myelin Stain)

2. Occipital pole
3. Interhemispheric fissure
34. Third ventricle
44. Hypothalamus
50. Mammillo-thalamic tract
58. Fimbria of fornix
59. Hippocampus
62. Lamina terminalis
63. Amygdala
64. Optic tract
65. Cerebral peduncle
67. Dentato-rubro-thalamic tract
68. Red nucleus
70. Medial leminiscus
73. Periaqueductal gray
74. Cerebral aqueduct
75. Superior colliculus
76. Parahippocampal gyrus
77. Inferior horn of lateral ventricle
78. Vermis of cerebellum
79. Substantia nigra
80. Spinothalamic tract
82. Reticular formation
84. Oculomotor nucleus (III)
85. Gyrus rectus
86. Olfactory sulcus
87. Olfactory trigone
88. Middle cerebral artery
89. Supraoptic commissure
90. Mammillary body
91. Interpeduncular cistern
92. Lateral leminiscus
93. Central tegmental tract

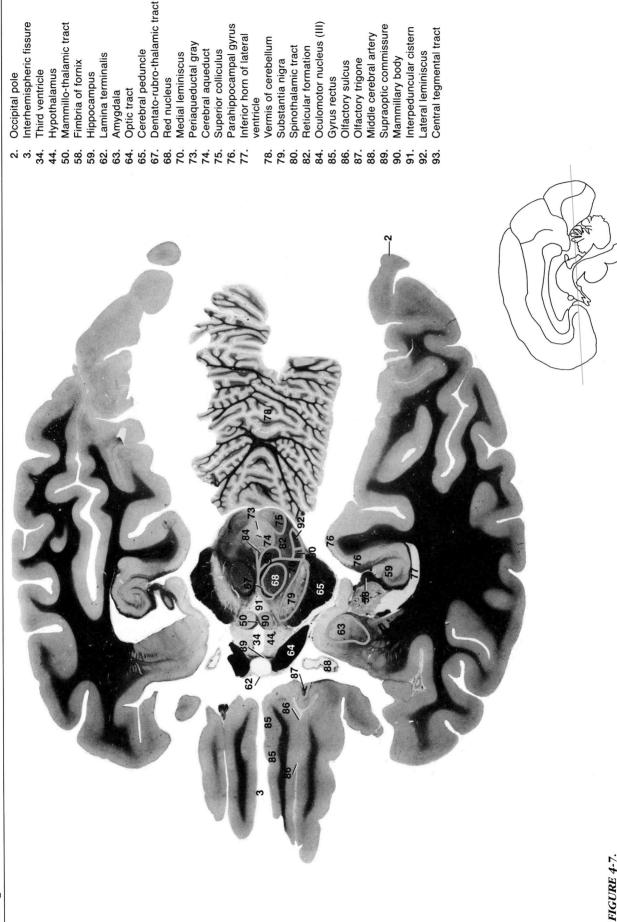

FIGURE 4-7.

Horizontal section through the base of the cerebrum, hypothalamus, and midbrain at the level of the supraoptic commissure, just inferior to section shown in Figure 4-6.

Horizontal Sections of the Brain (Myelin Stain)

34. Third ventricle
44. Hypothalamus
59. Hippocampus
63. Amygdala
65. Cerebral peduncle
68. Red nucleus
70. Medial leminiscus
73. Periaqueductal gray
74. Cerebral aqueduct
76. Parahippocampal gyrus
77. Inferior horn of lateral
     ventricle
78. Vermis of cerebellum
79. Substantia nigra
80. Spinothalamic tract
82. Reticular formation
87. Olfactory trigone
90. Mammillary body
93. Central tegmental tract
94. Optic chiasm
95. Medial longitudinal fasciculus
96. Trochlear nucleus (IV)

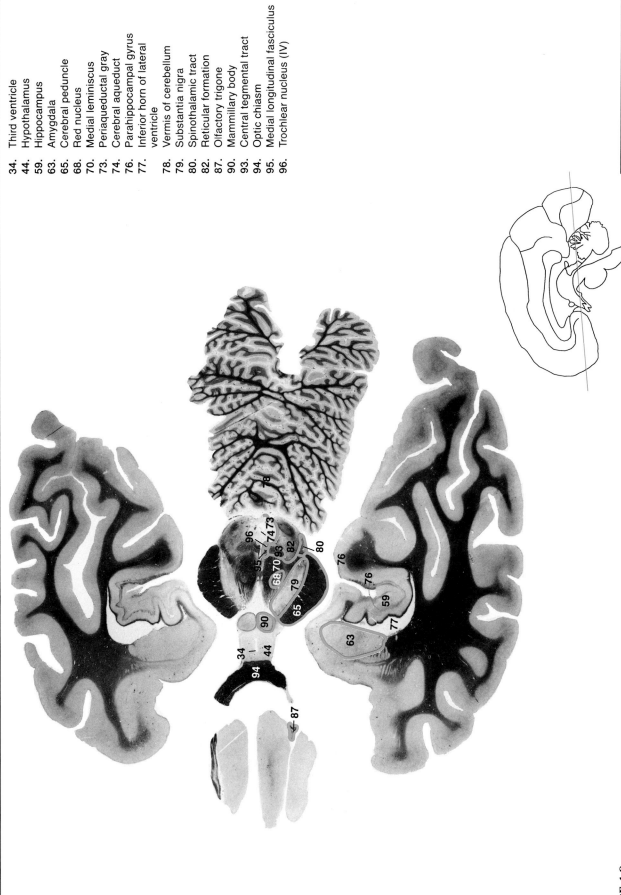

FIGURE 4-8.
Horizontal section through the optic chiasm.

63. Amygdala
65. Cerebral peduncle
70. Medial lemniscus
76. Parahippocampal gyrus
77. Inferior horn of lateral ventricle
78. Vermis of cerebellum
79. Substantia nigra
80. Spinothalamic tract
92. Lateral lemniscus
95. Medial longitudinal fasciculus
97. Superior cerebellar peduncle
98. Decussation of superior cerebellar peduncle
99. Fourth ventricle

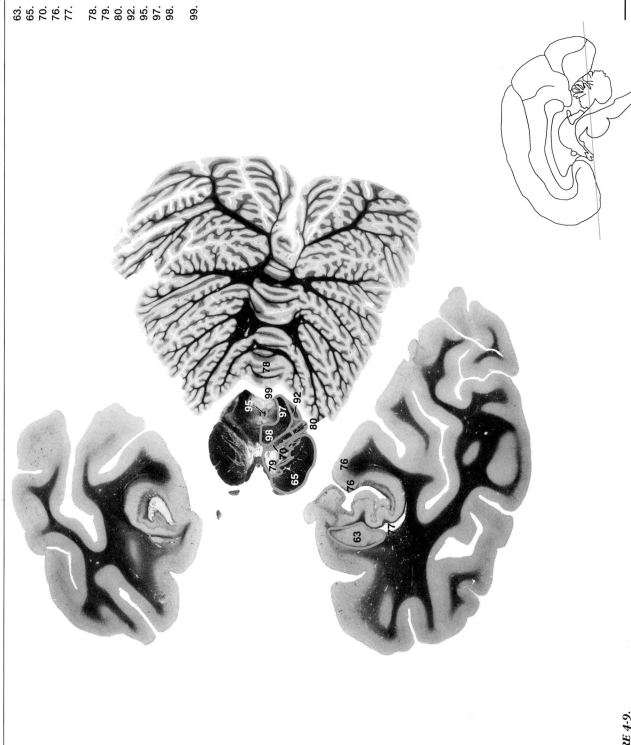

FIGURE 4-9.
Horizontal sections through the superior aspect of the fourth ventricle.

Atlas of the Human Brain, by Lothar Jennes, Harold H. Traurig, and P. Michael Conn. J. B. Lippincott Company, Philadelphia. © 1995.

The Brain Stem (Coronal Sections, Myelin Stain)

c h a p t e r

5

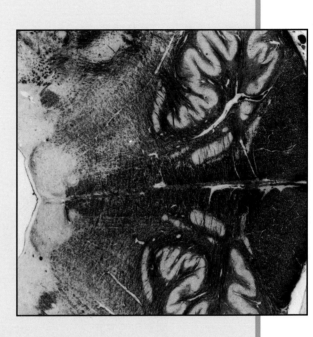

The Brain Stem (Coronal Sections, Myelin Stain)

1. Posterior median sulcus
2. Anterior median sulcus
3. Central gray of medulla
4. Pyramidal (motor) decussation
5. Pyramidal (motor) tract
6. Sensory decussation
7. Gracile fasciculus
8. Gracile nucleus
9. Cuneate fasciculus
10. Cuneate nucleus
11. Spinal trigeminal tract
12. Spinal trigeminal nucleus
13. Lateral reticular nucleus
14. Lateral and ventral spinothalamic and rubrospinal tracts
15. Reticulospinal, tectospinal, and vestibulospinal tracts
16. Spinocerebellar tracts

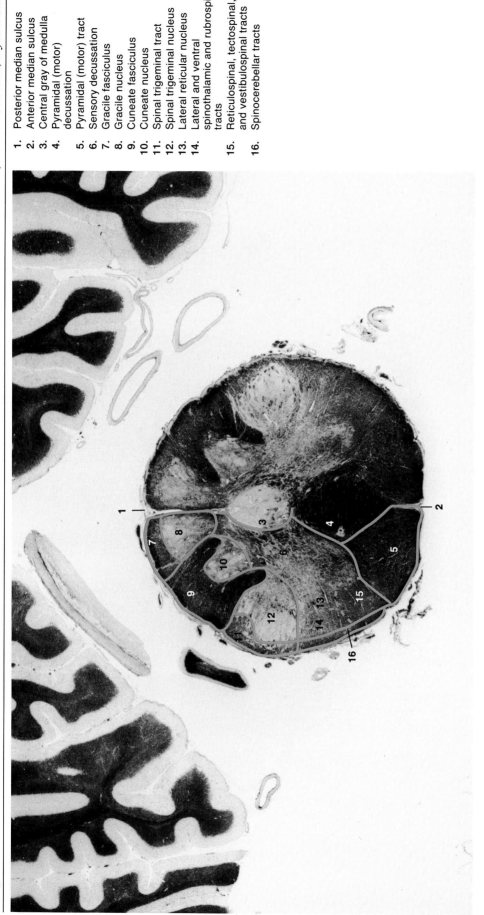

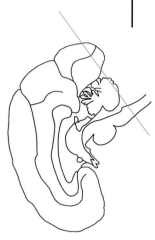

FIGURE 5-1.
Cross section of the caudal medulla at the level of the motor decussation.

1. Posterior median sulcus
2. Anterior median sulcus
3. Central gray of medulla
5. Pyramidal (motor) tract
6. Sensory decussation
7. Gracile fasciculus
8. Gracile nucleus
9. Cuneate fasciculus
10. Cuneate nucleus
11. Spinal trigeminal tract
12. Spinal trigeminal nucleus
13. Lateral reticular nucleus
14. Lateral and ventral
    spinothalamic and rubrospinal
    tracts
15. Reticulospinal, tectospinal,
    and vestibulospinal tracts
16. Spinocerebellar tracts
17. Medial longitudinal fasciculus
18. Tectospinal tract
19. Medial lemniscus
20. Accessory olive nuclei
21. Dorsal efferent vagus nucleus
22. Hypoglossal nucleus
23. Ventral trigeminothalamic tract
24. Ventral reticular nucleus
25. Nucleus ambiguus

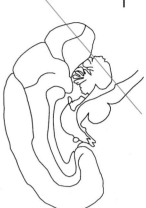

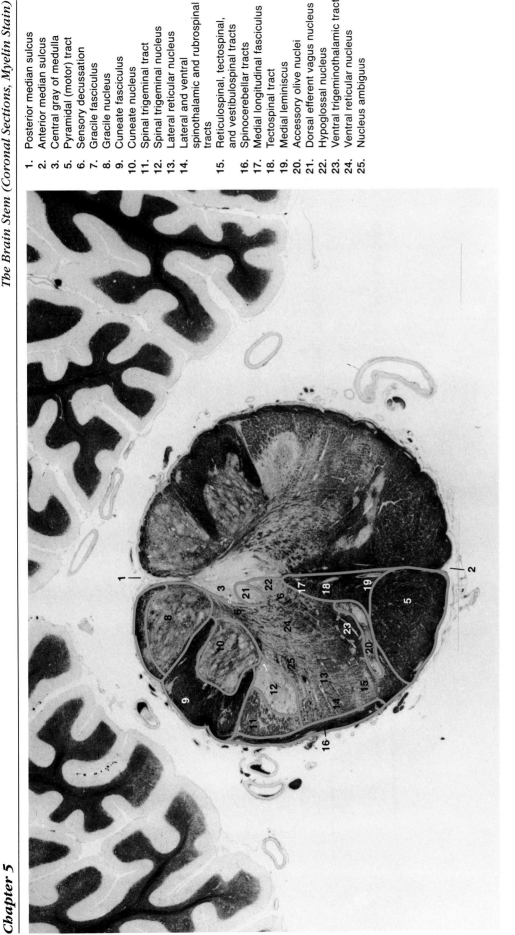

FIGURE 5-2.
Cross section of the caudal medulla at the level of the sensory decussation.

2. Anterior median sulcus
5. Pyramidal (motor) tract
7. Gracile fasciculus
8. Gracile nucleus
9. Cuneate fasciculus
10. Cuneate nucleus
11. Spinal trigeminal tract
12. Spinal trigeminal nucleus
13. Lateral reticular nucleus
14. Lateral and ventral
    spinothalamic and rubrospinal
    tracts
16. Spinocerebellar tracts
17. Medial longitudinal fasciculus
18. Tectospinal tract
19. Medial leminiscus
20. Accessory olive nuclei
22. Hypoglossal nucleus
24. Ventral reticular nucleus
25. Nucleus ambiguus
26. Dorsal vagus nucleus
27. Solitary fasciculus
28. Solitary nucleus
29. Central tegmental tract
30. Lateral cuneate nucleus
31. Arcuate nucleus
32. Paramedian reticular nucleus
33. Inferior olive nucleus
34. Area postrema
40. Olivocerebellar tract

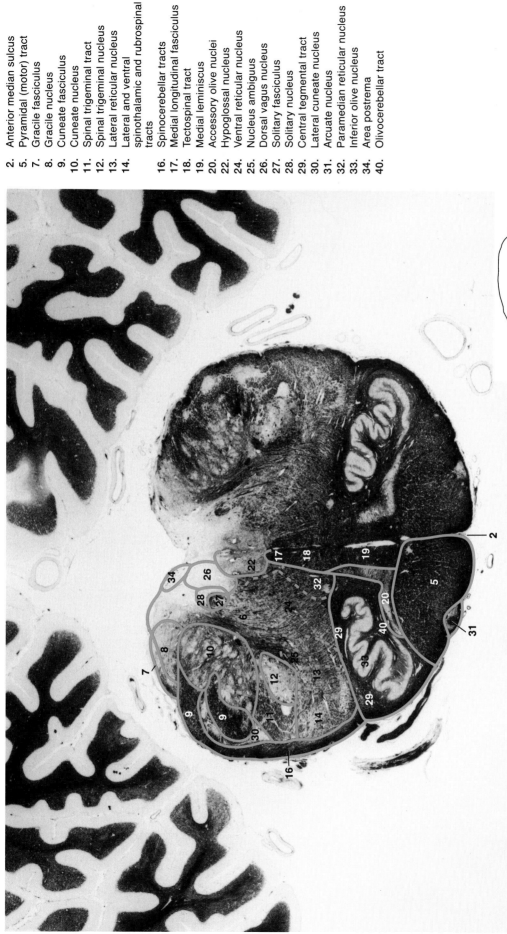

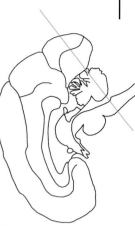

FIGURE 5-3.

Cross section of the mid-medulla at the level of the hypoglossal and vagal nuclei.

The Brain Stem (Coronal Sections, Myelin Stain)

2. Anterior median sulcus
5. Pyramidal (motor) tract
11. Spinal trigeminal tract
12. Spinal trigeminal nucleus
13. Lateral reticular nucleus
14. Lateral and ventral spinothalamic and rubrospinal tracts
17. Medial longitudinal fasciculus
18. Tectospinal tract
19. Medial lemniscus
20. Accessory olive nuclei
22. Hypoglossal nucleus
24. Ventral reticular nucleus
25. Nucleus ambiguus
26. Dorsal vagus nucleus
27. Solitary fasciculus
28. Solitary nucleus
29. Central tegmental tract
30. Lateral cuneate nucleus
32. Paramedian reticular nucleus
33. Inferior olive nucleus
34. Area postrema
35. Ventral spinocerebellar tract
36. Inferior cerebellar peduncle
37. Inferior vestibular nucleus
38. Medial vestibular nucleus
39. Dorsal longitudinal fasciculus
40. Olivocerebellar tract

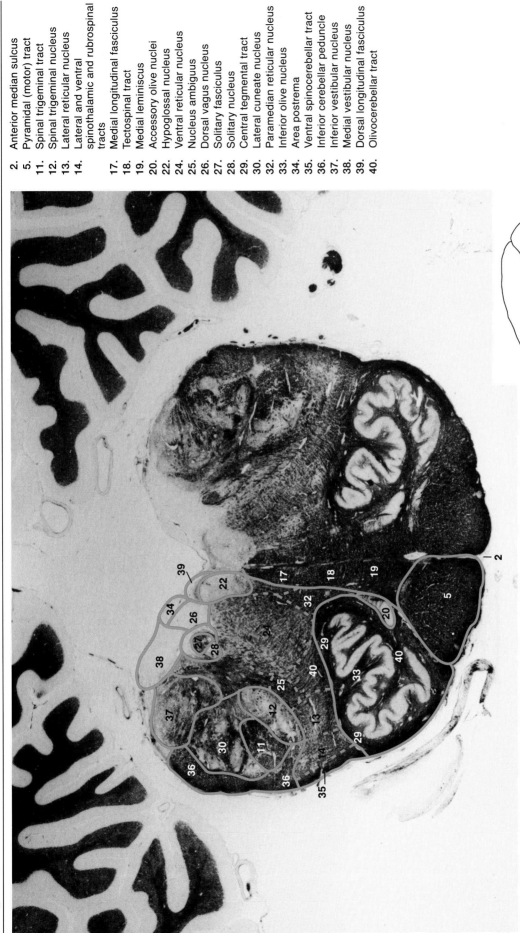

FIGURE 5-4.

Cross section of the mid-medulla at the level of the hypoglossal and vagal nuclei slightly superior to section shown in Figure 5-3.

2. Anterior median sulcus
5. Pyramidal (motor) tract
11. Spinal trigeminal tract
12. Spinal trigeminal nucleus
13. Lateral reticular nucleus
14. Lateral and ventral spinothalamic and rubrospinal tracts
17. Medial longitudinal fasciculus
18. Tectospinal tract
19. Medial lemniscus
20. Accessory olive nuclei
22. Hypoglossal nucleus
24. Ventral reticular nucleus
25. Nucleus ambiguus
27. Solitary fasciculus
28. Solitary nucleus
29. Central tegmental tract
30. Lateral cuneate nucleus
32. Paramedian reticular nucleus
33. Inferior olive nucleus
35. Ventral spinocerebellar tract
36. Inferior cerebellar peduncle
37. Inferior vestibular nucleus
38. Medial vestibular nucleus
39. Dorsal longitudinal fasciculus
40. Olivocerebellar tract
41. Nucleus raphe pallidus and obscuris
42. Parvicellular nucleus
43. Fourth ventricle
44. Choroid plexus of fourth ventricle
45. Posterior medullary velum

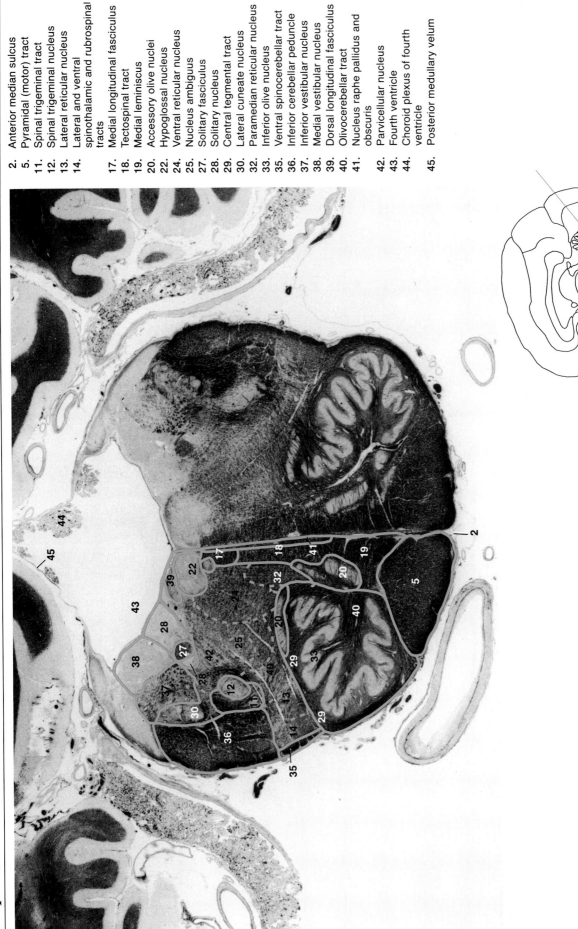

FIGURE 5-5.

Cross section of the mid-medulla at the level of the hypoglossal and vagal nuclei slightly superior to section shown in Figure 5-4.

2. Anterior median sulcus
5. Pyramidal (motor) tract
11. Spinal trigeminal tract
12. Spinal trigeminal nucleus
13. Lateral reticular nucleus
14. Lateral and ventral spinothalamic and rubrospinal tracts
17. Medial longitudinal fasciculus
18. Tectospinal tract
19. Medial leminiscus
20. Accessory olive nuclei
24. Ventral reticular nucleus
25. Nucleus ambiguus
27. Solitary fasciculus
28. Solitary nucleus
29. Central tegmental tract
32. Paramedian reticular nucleus
33. Inferior olive nucleus
35. Ventral spinocerebellar tract
36. Inferior cerebellar peduncle
37. Inferior vestibular nucleus
38. Medial vestibular nucleus
40. Olivocerebellar tract
41. Nucleus raphe pallidus and obscuris
42. Parvicellular nucleus
43. Fourth ventricle
44. Choroid plexus of fourth ventricle
46. Nucleus prepositus
47. Stria medullaris
48. Lateral aperture of Luschka
49. Glossopharyngeal nerve (IX)

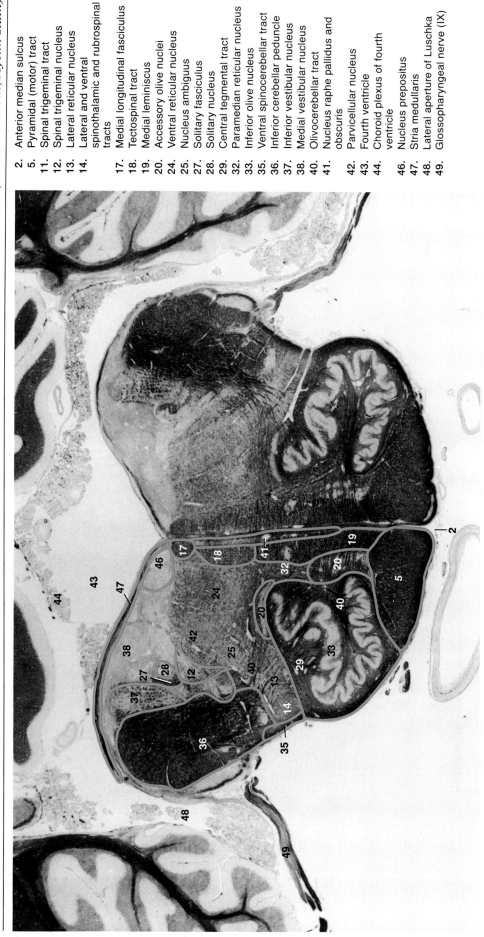

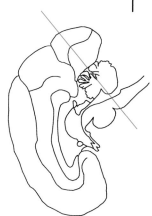

FIGURE 5-6.

Cross section of the rostral medulla at the level of the glossopharyngeal nuclei.

The Brain Stem (Coronal Sections, Myelin Stain)

2. Anterior median sulcus
5. Pyramidal (motor) tract
11. Spinal trigeminal tract
12. Spinal trigeminal nucleus
13. Lateral reticular nucleus
14. Lateral and ventral spinothalamic and rubrospinal tracts
17. Medial longitudinal fasciculus
18. Tectospinal tract
19. Medial lemniscus
20. Accessory olive nuclei
27. Solitary fasciculus
28. Solitary nucleus
29. Central tegmental tract
32. Paramedian reticular nucleus
33. Inferior olive nucleus
35. Ventral spinocerebellar tract
36. Inferior cerebellar peduncle
37. Inferior vestibular nucleus
38. Medial vestibular nucleus
40. Olivocerebellar tract
41. Nucleus raphe pallidus and obscuris
42. Parvicellular nucleus
43. Fourth ventricle
44. Choroid plexus of fourth ventricle
46. Nucleus prepositus
47. Stria medullaris
49. Glossopharyngeal nerve (IX)
50. Nodulus of cerebellum
51. Dorsal cochlear nucleus
52. Ventral cochlear nucleus
53. Rubrospinal tract
54. Gigantocellular nucleus
55. Ventral paraflocculus
56. Dentate nucleus
57. Inferior salivatory nucleus

58

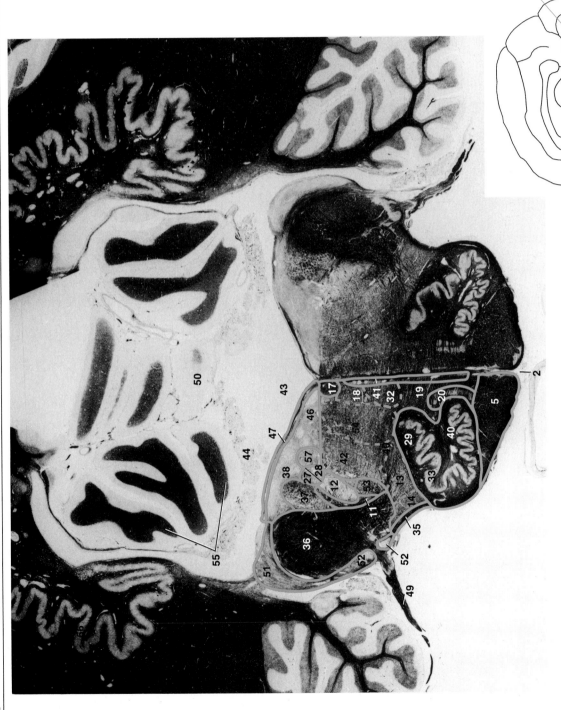

FIGURE 5-7.

Cross section of the rostral medulla at the level of the glossopharyngeal nuclei slightly superior to section shown in Figure 5-6.

The Brain Stem (Coronal Sections, Myelin Stain)

2. Anterior median sulcus
5. Pyramidal (motor) tract
11. Spinal trigeminal tract
12. Spinal trigeminal nucleus
14. Lateral and ventral spinothalamic and rubrospinal tracts
17. Medial longitudinal fasciculus
18. Tectospinal tract
19. Medial lemniscus
29. Central tegmental tract
31. Arcuate nucleus
35. Ventral spinocerebellar tract
36. Inferior cerebellar peduncle
38. Medial vestibular nucleus
39. Dorsal longitudinal fascicle
41. Nucleus raphe pallidus and obscuris
42. Parvicellular nucleus
43. Fourth ventricle
50. Nodulus of cerebellum
52. Ventral cochlear nucleus
54. Gigantocellular nucleus
56. Dentate nucleus
58. Facial nucleus
59. Reticulotegmental nucleus
60. Internal genu of facial nerve (VII)
61. Abducens nucleus
62. Lateral vestibular nucleus
63. Superior vestibular nucleus
64. Superior cerebellar peduncle
65. Emboliform nucleus
66. Globose nucleus
67. Fastigial nucleus
68. Middle cerebellar peduncle
69. Facial nerve (VII)
70. Roots of vestibulocochlear nerve (VIII)
71. Trapezoid fibers
72. Superior olive nucleus

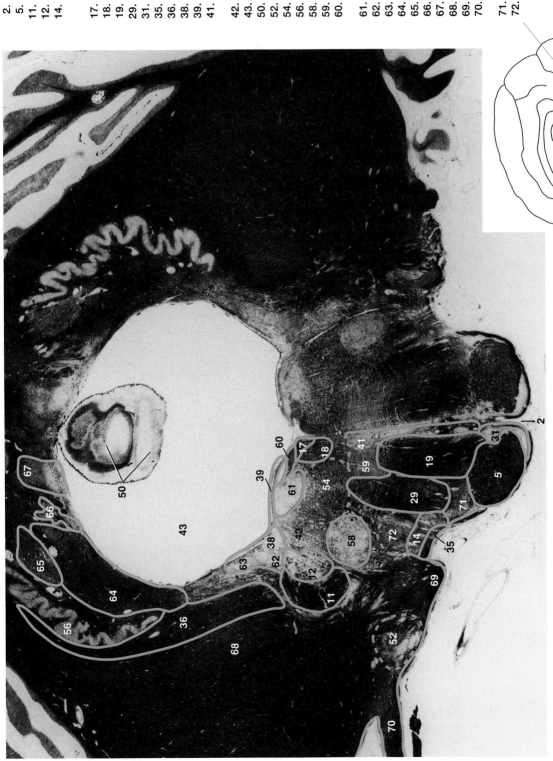

FIGURE 5-8.

Cross section of the brain stem at the junction of the medulla and pons at the level of the roots of the fascial (VII) and vestibulocochlear (VIII) nerves.

The Brain Stem (Coronal Sections, Myelin Stain)

2. Anterior median sulcus
5. Pyramidal (motor) tract
11. Spinal trigeminal tract
12. Spinal trigeminal nucleus
17. Medial longitudinal fasciculus
18. Tectospinal tract
19. Medial lemniscus
27. Solitary fasciculus
28. Solitary nucleus
29. Central tegmental tract
31. Arcuate nucleus
36. Inferior cerebellar peduncle
38. Medial vestibular nucleus
39. Dorsal longitudinal fascicle
42. Parvicellular nucleus
43. Fourth ventricle
52. Ventral cochlear nucleus
53. Rubrospinal tract
54. Gigantocellular nucleus
56. Dentate nucleus
58. Facial nucleus
59. Reticulotegmental nucleus
60. Internal genu of facial nerve (VII)
61. Abducens nucleus
62. Lateral vestibular nucleus
63. Superior vestibular nucleus
64. Superior cerebellar peduncle
65. Emboliform nucleus
66. Globose nucleus
67. Fastigial nucleus
68. Middle cerebellar peduncle
69. Facial nerve (VII)
70. Roots of vestibulocochlear nerve (VIII)
71. Trapezoid fibers
72. Superior olive nucleus
73. Pontine nuclei
74. Pontocerebellar tract
75. Superior salivatory nucleus
76. Raphe magnus nucleus
77. Paramedian pontine reticular formation
78. Roots of abducens nerve (VI)

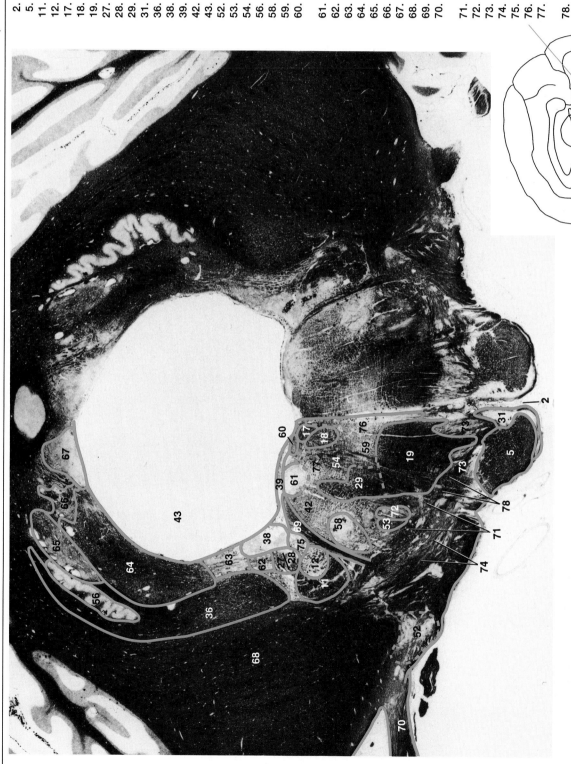

60

FIGURE 5-9.
Cross section of the caudal pons at the level of the facial motor and abducens nuclei.

2. Anterior median sulcus
5. Pyramidal (motor) tract
11. Spinal trigeminal tract
12. Spinal trigeminal nucleus
17. Medial longitudinal fasciculus
18. Tectospinal tract
19. Medial lemniscus
27. Solitary fasciculus
28. Solitary nucleus
29. Central tegmental tract
31. Arcuate nucleus
36. Inferior cerebellar peduncle
38. Medial vestibular nucleus
39. Dorsal longitudinal fascicle
42. Parvicellular nucleus
43. Fourth ventricle
52. Ventral cochlear nucleus
58. Facial nucleus
59. Reticulotegmental nucleus
60. Internal genu of facial nerve (VII)
61. Abducens nucleus
62. Lateral vestibular nucleus
63. Superior vestibular nucleus
64. Superior cerebellar peduncle
65. Emboliform nucleus
66. Globose nucleus
67. Fastigial nucleus
68. Middle cerebellar peduncle
69. Facial nerve (VII)
70. Roots of vestibulocochlear nerve (VIII)
72. Superior olive nucleus
73. Pontine nuclei
74. Pontocerebellar tract
75. Superior salivatory nucleus
76. Raphe magnus nucleus
77. Paramedian pontine reticular formation
78. Roots of abducens nerve (VI)
87. Lateral lemniscus
88. Spinothalamic tracts

61

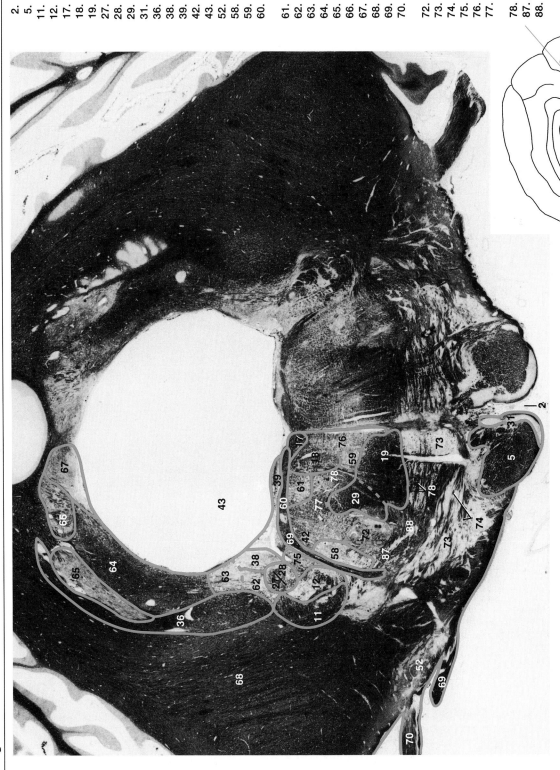

FIGURE 5-10.

Cross section of the caudal pons at the level of the fascial motor and abducens nuclei and the internal genu of the fascial nerve just superior to section shown in Figure 5-9.

2. Anterior median sulcus
5. Pyramidal (motor) tract
17. Medial longitudinal fasciculus
18. Tectospinal tract
19. Medial leminiscus
29. Central tegmental tract
31. Arcuate nucleus
35. Ventral spinocerebellar tract
39. Dorsal longitudinal fascicle
43. Fourth ventricle
59. Reticulotegmental nucleus
63. Superior vestibular nucleus
64. Superior cerebellar peduncle
68. Middle cerebellar peduncle
72. Superior olive nucleus
73. Pontine nuclei
74. Pontocerebellar tract
79. Central pontine reticular nucleus
80. Motor nucleus of trigeminal nerve (V)
81. Mesencephalic trigeminal tract
82. Mesencephalic trigeminal nucleus
83. Principal sensory trigeminal nucleus
84. Lingula of cerebellum
85. Root of trigeminal nerve (V)
87. Lateral leminiscus
88. Spinothalamic tracts
89. Periaqueductal central gray
90. Superior medullary velum
91. Central nucleus of raphe, pars superior
94. Parabrachial nucleus

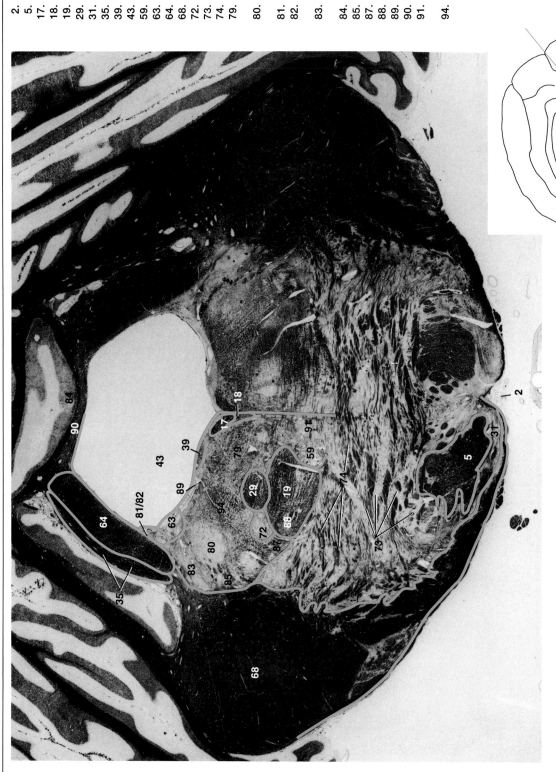

FIGURE 5-11.
Cross section of the mid pons at the level of the trigeminal nuclei.

5. Pyramidal (motor) tract
17. Medial longitudinal fasciculus
18. Tectospinal tract
19. Medial leminiscus
23. Ventral trigeminothalamic tract
29. Central tegmental tract
35. Ventral spinocerebellar tract
39. Dorsal longitudinal fascicle
43. Fourth ventricle
53. Rubrospinal tract
59. Reticulotegmental nucleus
63. Superior vestibular nucleus
64. Superior cerebellar peduncle
68. Middle cerebellar peduncle
72. Superior olive nucleus
73. Pontine nuclei
74. Pontocerebellar tract
79. Central pontine reticular nucleus
80. Motor nucleus of trigeminal nerve (V)
81. Mesencephalic trigeminal tract
82. Mesencephalic trigeminal nucleus
83. Principal sensory trigeminal nucleus
84. Lingula of cerebellum
85. Root of trigeminal nerve (V)
86. Locus ceruleus
87. Lateral leminiscus
88. Spinothalamic tracts
89. Periaqueductal central gray
90. Superior medullary velum
91. Central nucleus of raphe, pars superior
94. Parabrachial nucleus

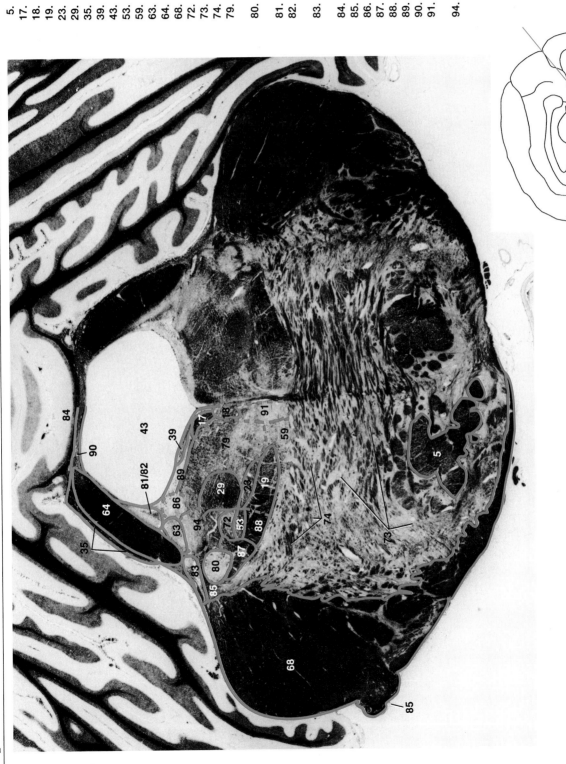

FIGURE 5-12.

Cross section of the mid pons at the level of the trigeminal nuclei just superior to section shown in Figure 5-11.

5. Pyramidal (motor) tract
17. Medial longitudinal fasciculus
19. Medial leminiscus
23. Ventral trigeminothalamic tract
29. Central tegmental tract
53. Rubrospinal tract
59. Reticulotegmental nucleus
64. Superior cerebellar peduncle
68. Middle cerebellar peduncle
73. Pontine nuclei
74. Pontocerebellar tract
79. Central pontine reticular
    nucleus
81. Mesencephalic trigeminal tract
86. Locus ceruleus
87. Lateral leminiscus
88. Spinothalamic tracts
89. Periaqueductal central gray
91. Central nucleus of raphe, pars
    superior
92. Dorsal nucleus of raphe
93. Decussation of trochlear
    nerve
94. Parabrachial nucleus
95. Fronto-pontine tract
96. Occipito-temporo-pontine tract
97. Dorsal trigeminothalamic tract
99. Cerebral aqueduct

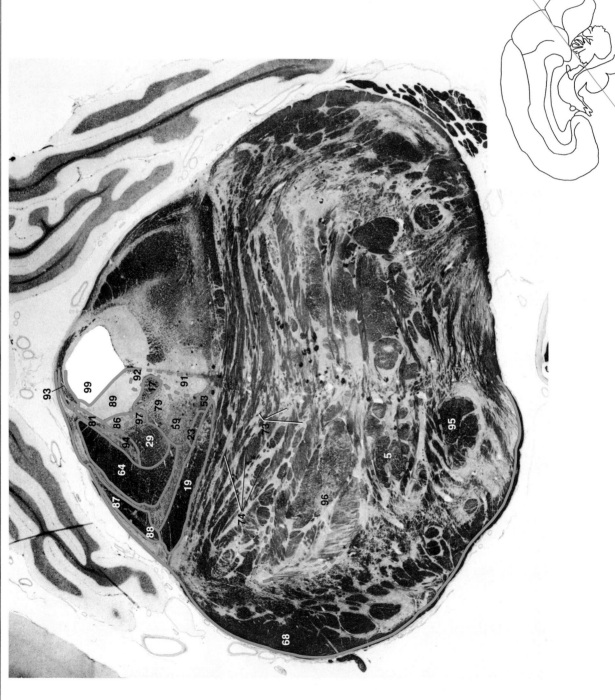

FIGURE 5-13.
Cross section of the rostral pons.

17. Medial longitudinal fasciculus
18. Tectospinal tract
19. Medial leminiscus
23. Ventral trigeminothalamic tract
29. Central tegmental tract
53. Rubrospinal tract
59. Reticulotegmental nucleus
73. Pontine nuclei
74. Pontocerebellar tract
79. Central pontine reticular nucleus
81. Mesencephalic trigeminal tract
82. Mesencephalic trigeminal nucleus
87. Lateral leminiscus
88. Spinothalamic tracts
89. Periaqueductal central gray
91. Central nucleus of raphe, pars superior
92. Dorsal nucleus of raphe
94. Parabrachial nucleus
98. Spinotectal tract
99. Cerebral aqueduct
100. Trochlear nucleus
101. Interpeduncular nucleus
102. Commissure of inferior colliculus
103. Nucleus of inferior colliculus
104. Brachium of inferior colliculus
105. Decussation of cerebellar peduncle

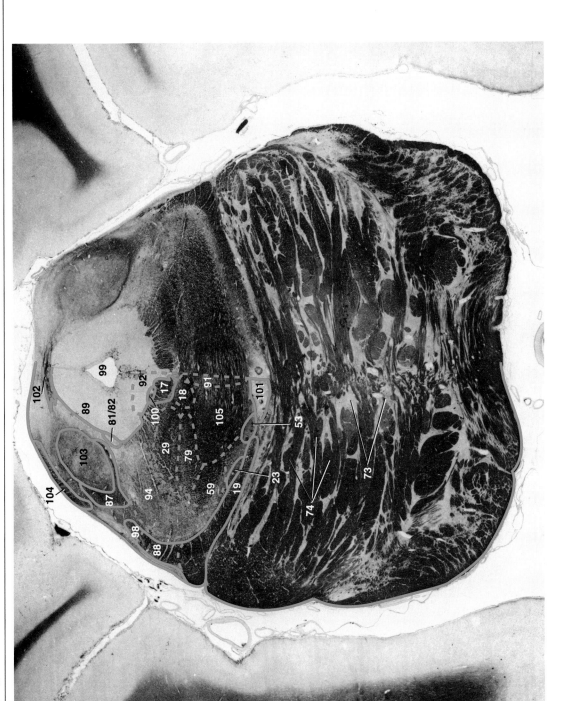

FIGURE 5-14.
Cross section of the caudal midbrain at the level of the inferior colliculus.

5. Pyramidal (motor) tract
17. Medial longitudinal fasciculus
19. Medial leminiscus
23. Ventral trigeminothalamic tract
29. Central tegmental tract
53. Rubrospinal tract
59. Reticulotegmental nucleus
68. Middle cerebellar peduncle
73. Pontine nuclei
74. Pontocerebellar tract
79. Central pontine reticular nucleus
81. Mesencephalic trigeminal tract
82. Mesencephalic trigeminal nucleus
88. Spinothalamic tracts
89. Periaqueductal central gray
91. Central nucleus of raphe, pars superior
92. Dorsal nucleus of raphe
94. Parabrachial nucleus
95. Frontopontine tract
96. Occipito-temporo-pontine tract
97. Dorsal trigeminothalamic tract
98. Spinotectal tract
99. Cerebral aqueduct
100. Trochlear nucleus
101. Interpeduncular nucleus
104. Brachium of inferior colliculus
105. Decussation of cerebellar peduncle
106. Nigrostriatal tract
107. Cerebral peduncle
113. Commissure of superior colliculus
114. Superior colliculus
115. Pedunculopontine nucleus
116. Substantia nigra

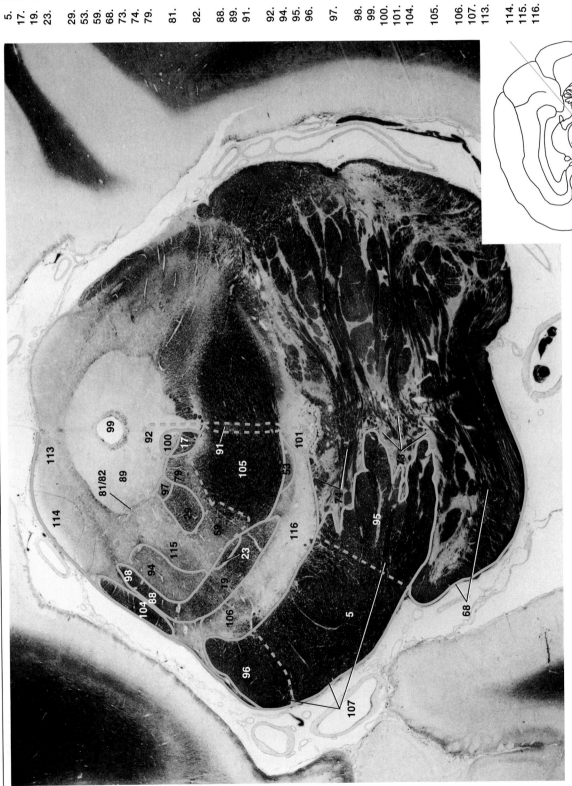

FIGURE 5-15.
Cross section of the caudal midbrain at the level of the trochlear nucleus.

5. Pyramidal (motor) tract
17. Medial longitudinal fasciculus
19. Medial leminiscus
23. Ventral trigeminothalamic tract
29. Central tegmental tract
59. Reticulotegmental nucleus
79. Central pontine reticular nucleus
81. Mesencephalic trigeminal tract
82. Mesencephalic trigeminal nucleus
88. Spinothalamic tracts
89. Periaqueductal central gray
91. Central nucleus of raphe, pars superior
92. Dorsal nucleus of raphe
94. Parabrachial nucleus
95. Frontopontine tract
96. Occipito-temporo-pontine tract
97. Dorsal trigeminothalamic tract
99. Cerebral aqueduct
100. Trochlear nucleus
101. Interpeduncular nucleus
104. Brachium of inferior colliculus
105. Decussation of cerebellar peduncle
106. Nigrostriatal tract
107. Cerebral peduncle
108. Oculomotor nucleus
109. Tegmental area
110. Medial geniculate body
111. Posterior cerebral artery
112. Interpeduncular cistern
113. Commissure of superior colliculus
114. Superior colliculus
115. Pedunculo-pontine nucleus
116. Substantia nigra

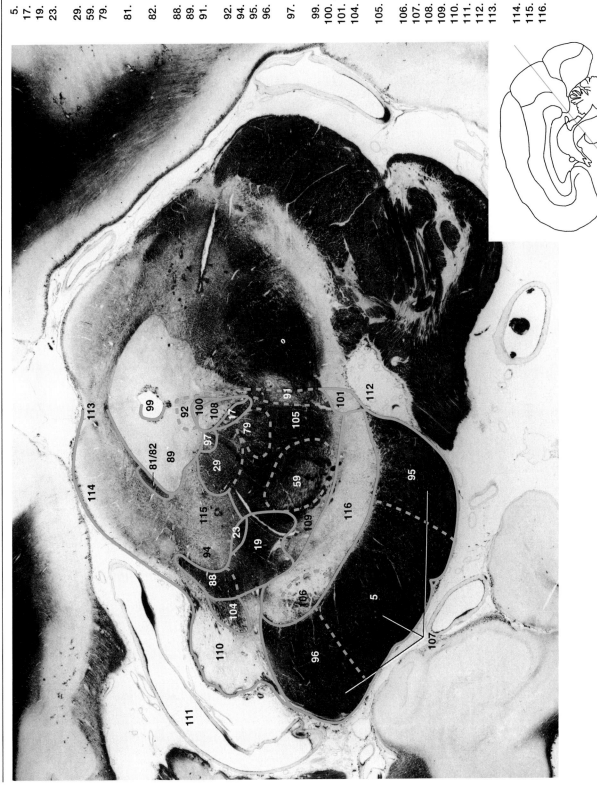

FIGURE 5-16.
Cross section of the caudal midbrain at the level of the superior colliculus.

67

The Brain Stem (Coronal Sections, Myelin Stain)

5. Pyramidal (motor) tract
17. Medial longitudinal fasciculus
19. Medial lemniscus
23. Ventral trigeminothalamic tract
29. Central tegmental tract
53. Rubrospinal tract
88. Spinothalamic tracts
89. Periaqueductal central gray
95. Frontopontine tract
96. Occipito-temporo-pontine tract
99. Cerebral aqueduct
101. Interpeduncular nucleus
104. Brachium of inferior colliculus
106. Nigrostriatal tract
107. Cerebral peduncle
109. Tegmental area
110. Medial geniculate body
112. Interpeduncular cistern
114. Superior colliculus
116. Substantia nigra
117. Pulvinar
118. Brachium of superior colliculus
119. Peripeduncular nucleus
120. Oculomotor nerve (III)
121. Fasciculus retroflexus
122. Nucleus linearis
123. Prerubral tract
124. Nucleus cuneiformis
125. Reticular formation
126. Pretectal area
127. Nucleus of Darkschewitsch
128. Nucleus of Cajal
129. Lateral geniculate nucleus
131. Cerebello-rubro-thalamic tract
133. Red nucleus
134. Corpus callosum
135. Quadrigeminal cistern
136. Commissure of superior colliculus
137. Posterior commissure

68

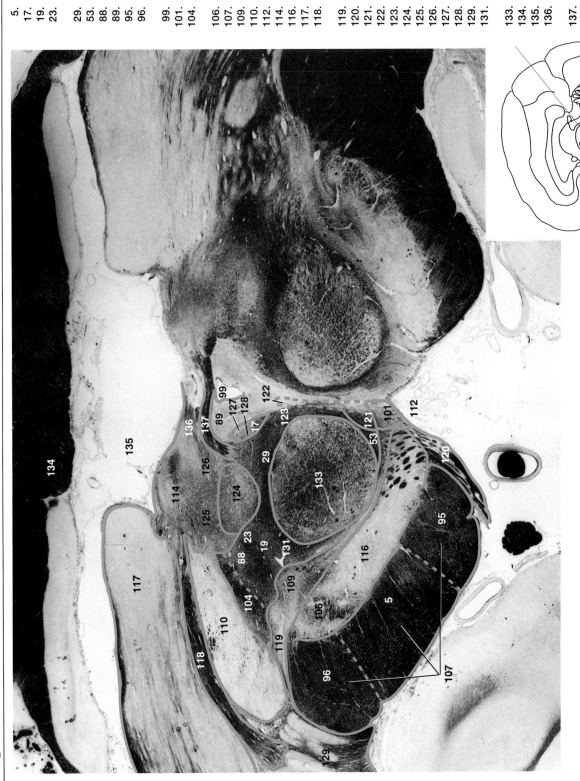

FIGURE 5-17.
Cross section of the rostral midbrain at the level of the red nucleus and the superior colliculus.

The Brain Stem (Coronal Sections, Myelin Stain)

5. Pyramidal (motor) tract
17. Medial longitudinal fasciculus
19. Medial leminiscus
23. Ventral trigeminothalamic tract
29. Central tegmental tract
53. Rubrospinal tract
88. Spinothalamic tracts
89. Periaqueductal central gray
95. Frontopontine tract
96. Occipito-temporo-pontine tract
99. Cerebral aqueduct
101. Interpeduncular nucleus
104. Brachium of inferior colliculus
106. Nigrostriatal tract
107. Cerebral peduncle
109. Tegmental area
110. Medial geniculate body
112. Interpeduncular cistern
114. Superior colliculus
116. Substantia nigra
117. Pulvinar
119. Peripeduncular nucleus
120. Oculomotor nerve (III)
121. Fasciculus retroflexus
122. Nucleus linearis
123. Prerubral tract
124. Nucleus cuneiformis
125. Reticular formation
126. Pretectal area
127. Nucleus of Darkschewitch
128. Nucleus of Cajal
129. Lateral geniculate nucleus
130. Subthalamus
131. Cerebello-rubro-thalamic tract
133. Red nucleus
134. Corpus callosum
135. Quadrigeminal cistern
137. Posterior commissure

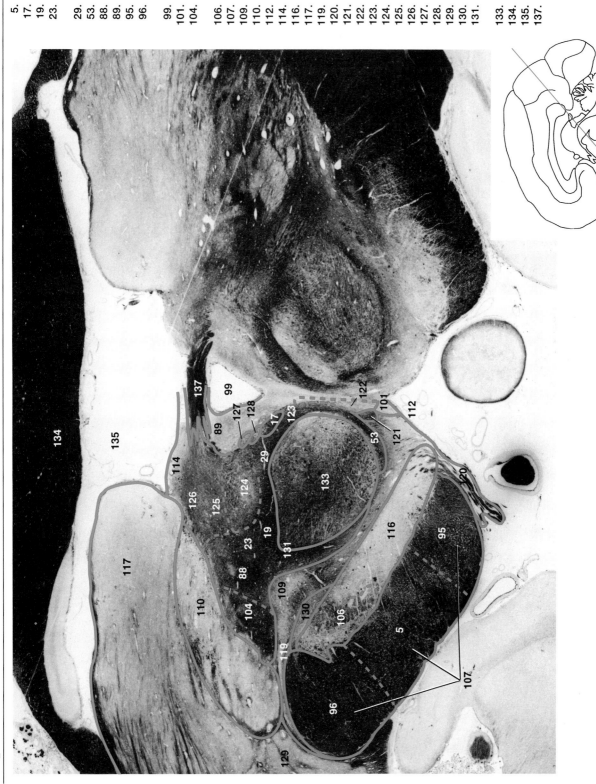

FIGURE 5-18.
Cross section of the rostral midbrain at the level of the posterior commissure.

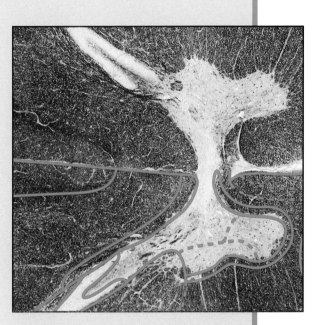

Atlas of the Human Brain, by Lothar Jennes,
Harold H. Traurig, and P. Michael Conn.
J. B. Lippincott Company, Philadelphia, © 1995.

The Spinal Cord (Coronal Sections, Myelin Stain)

c h a p t e r 6

1. Gracile fasciculus
3. Ventral white commissure
4. Dorsal median sulcus
5. Ventral median fissure
6. Substantia gelatinosa
7. Nucleus proprius
8. Lateral motor nuclei
9. Propriospinal tract
10. Medial motor nuclei
11. Dorsolateral tract (Lissauer's fascicle)
12. Lateral corticospinal tract
13. Ventral spinothalamic tract
15. Ventral corticospinal tract
16. Central canal
19. Ventral spinocerebellar tract
24. Lateral spinothalamic and spinotectal tracts

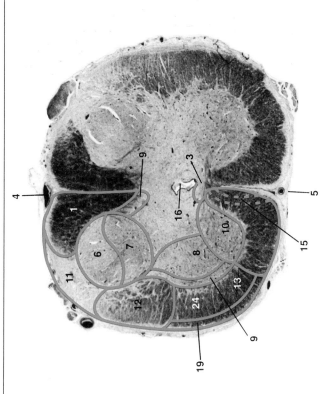

FIGURE 6-1.

Transverse section through the lower sacral spinal cord (S4).

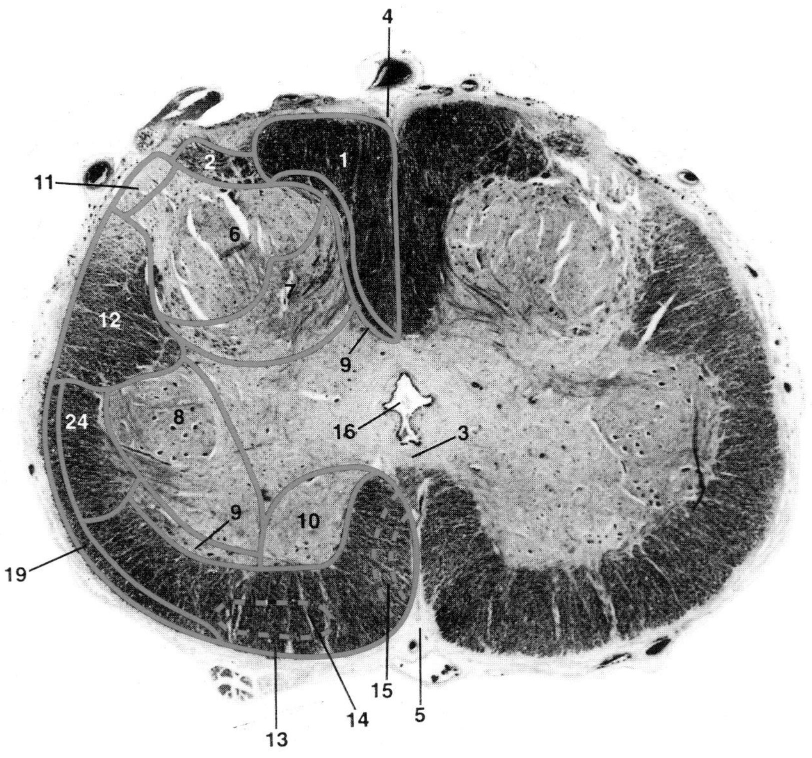

The Spinal Cord (Coronal Sections, Myelin Stain)

1. Gracile fasciculus
2. Dorsal root of spinal nerve
3. Ventral white commissure
4. Dorsal median sulcus
5. Ventral median fissure
6. Substantia gelatinosa
7. Nucleus proprius
8. Lateral motor nuclei
9. Propriospinal tract
10. Medial motor nuclei
11. Dorsolateral tract (Lissauer's fascicle)
12. Lateral corticospinal tract
13. Ventral spinothalamic tract
14. Lateral vestibulospinal tract
15. Ventral corticospinal tract
16. Central canal
19. Ventral spinocerebellar tract
24. Lateral spinothalamic and spinotectal tracts

FIGURE 6-2.
Transverse section through the upper sacral spinal cord (S2).

The Spinal Cord (Coronal Sections, Myelin Stain)

1. Gracile fasciculus
2. Dorsal root of spinal nerve
3. Ventral white commissure
4. Dorsal median sulcus
5. Ventral median fissure
6. Substantia gelatinosa
7. Nucleus proprius
8. Lateral motor nuclei
9. Propriospinal tract
10. Medial motor nuclei
11. Dorsolateral tract (Lissauer's fascicle)
12. Lateral corticospinal tract
13. Ventral spinothalamic tract
14. Lateral vestibulospinal tract
15. Ventral corticospinal tract
16. Central canal
19. Ventral spinocerebellar tract
24. Lateral spinothalamic and spinotectal tracts

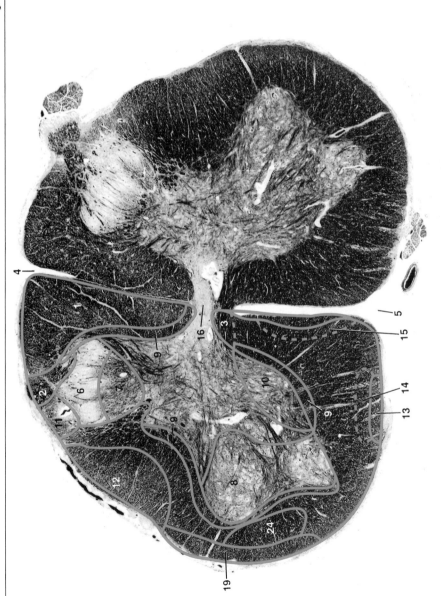

FIGURE 6-3.
Transverse section through the lower lumbar spinal cord (L4).

The Spinal Cord (Coronal Sections, Myelin Stain)

1. Gracile fasciculus
3. Ventral white commissure
4. Dorsal median sulcus
5. Ventral median fissure
6. Substantia gelatinosa
7. Nucleus proprius
9. Propriospinal tract
10. Medial motor nuclei
11. Dorsolateral tract (Lissauer's fascicle)
12. Lateral corticospinal tract
13. Ventral spinothalamic tract
14. Lateral vestibulospinal tract
15. Ventral corticospinal tract
16. Central canal
17. Nucleus dorsalis (Clarke)
18. Dorsal spinocerebellar tract
19. Ventral spinocerebellar tract
22. Intermediolateral nucleus
24. Lateral spinothalamic and spinotectal tracts
25. Rubrospinal tract

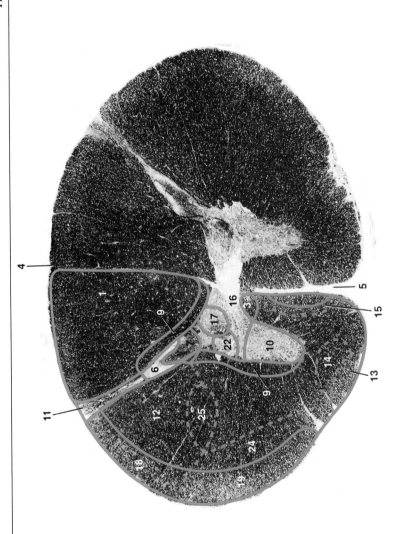

FIGURE 6-4.
Transverse section through the lower thoracic spinal cord (T11).

The Spinal Cord (Coronal Sections, Myelin Stain)

1. Gracile fasciculus
3. Ventral white commissure
4. Dorsal median sulcus
5. Ventral median fissure
6. Substantia gelatinosa
7. Nucleus proprius
9. Propriospinal tract
10. Medial motor nuclei
11. Dorsolateral tract (Lissauer's fascicle)
12. Lateral corticospinal tract
13. Ventral spinothalamic tract
14. Lateral vestibulospinal tract
15. Ventral corticospinal tract
16. Central canal
17. Nucleus dorsalis (Clarke)
18. Dorsal spinocerebellar tract
19. Ventral spinocerebellar tract
22. Intermediolateral nucleus
23. Cuneate fasciculus
24. Lateral spinothalamic and spinotectal tracts
25. Rubrospinal tract

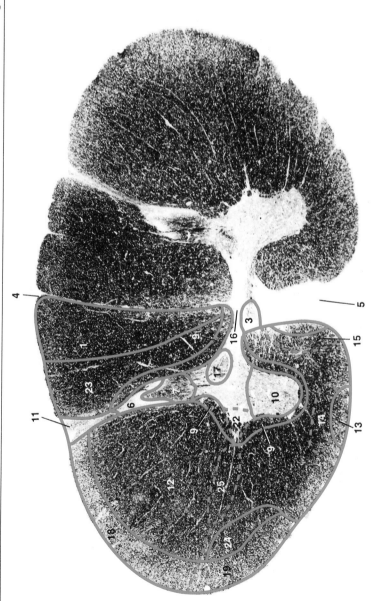

FIGURE 6-5.
Transverse section through the upper thoracic spinal cord (T2).

The Spinal Cord (Coronal Sections, Myelin Stain)

1. Gracile fasciculus
3. Ventral white commissure
4. Dorsal median sulcus
5. Ventral median fissure
6. Substantia gelatinosa
7. Nucleus proprius
8. Lateral motor nucleus
9. Propriospinal tract
10. Medial motor nuclei
11. Dorsolateral tract (Lissauer's fascicle)
12. Lateral corticospinal tract
13. Ventral spinothalamic tract
14. Lateral vestibulospinal tract
15. Ventral corticospinal tract
16. Central canal
18. Dorsal spinocerebellar tract
19. Ventral spinocerebellar tract
20. Dorsal intermediate sulcus
23. Cuneate fasciculus
24. Lateral spinothalamic and spinotectal tracts
25. Rubrospinal tract

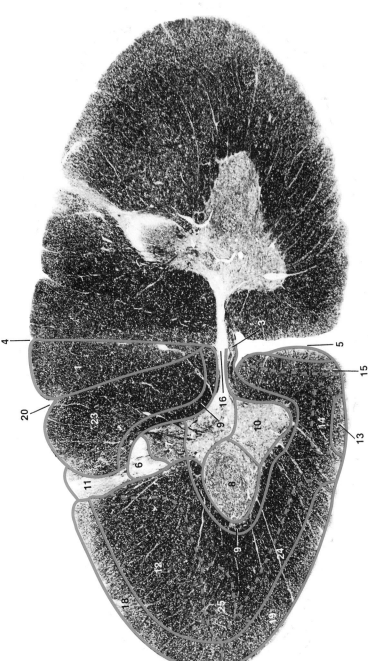

FIGURE 6-6.
Transverse section through the lower cervical spinal cord (C8).

The Spinal Cord (Coronal Sections, Myelin Stain)

1. Gracile fasciculus
3. Ventral white commissure
4. Dorsal median sulcus
5. Ventral median fissure
6. Substantia gelatinosa
7. Nucleus proprius
8. Lateral motor nucleus
9. Propriospinal tract
10. Medial motor nuclei
11. Dorsolateral tract (Lissauer's fascicle)
12. Lateral corticospinal tract
13. Ventral spinothalamic tract
14. Lateral vestibulospinal tract
15. Ventral corticospinal tract
16. Central canal
18. Dorsal spinocerebellar tract
19. Ventral spinocerebellar tract
20. Dorsal intermediate sulcus
23. Cuneate fasciculus
24. Lateral spinothalamic and spinotectal tracts
25. Rubrospinal tract

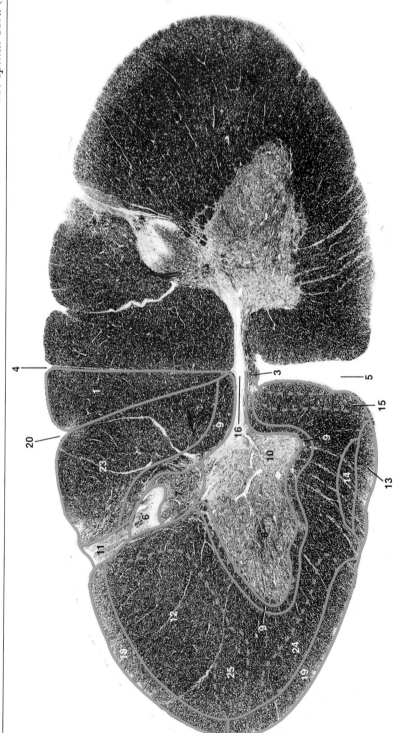

FIGURE 6-7.
Transverse section through the lower cervical spinal cord (C7).

The Spinal Cord (Coronal Sections, Myelin Stain)

1. Gracile fasciculus
3. Ventral white commissure
4. Dorsal median sulcus
5. Ventral median fissure
6. Substantia gelatinosa
7. Nucleus proprius
9. Propriospinal tract
10. Medial motor nuclei
11. Dorsolateral tract (Lissauer's fascicle)
12. Lateral corticospinal tract
13. Ventral spinothalamic tract
14. Lateral vestibulospinal tract
15. Ventral corticospinal tract
16. Central canal
18. Dorsal spinocerebellar tract
19. Ventral spinocerebellar tract
20. Dorsal intermediate sulcus
21. Accessory nucleus (XI)
23. Cuneate fasciculus
24. Lateral spinothalamic and spinotectal tracts
25. Rubrospinal tract

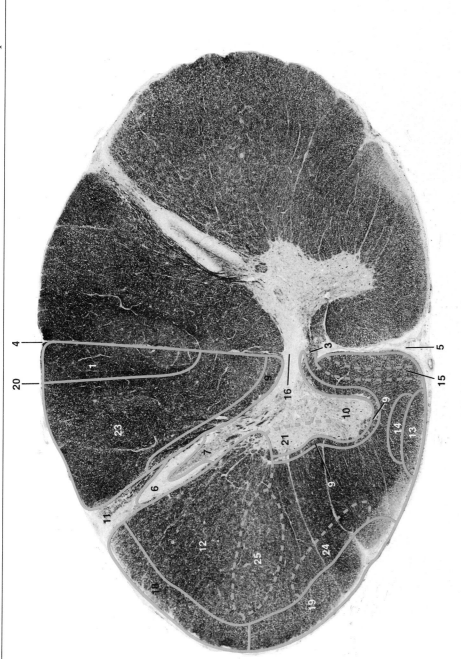

FIGURE 6-8.

Transverse section through the upper cervical spinal cord (C2).

The Spinal Cord (Coronal Sections, Myelin Stain)

1. Gracile fasciculus
2. Dorsal root of spinal nerve
3. Ventral white commissure
4. Dorsal median sulcus
5. Ventral median fissure
6. Substantia gelatinosa
7. Nucleus proprius
9. Propriospinal tract
10. Medial motor nuclei
11. Dorsolateral tract (Lissauer's fascicle)
12. Lateral corticospinal tract
13. Ventral spinothalamic tract
14. Lateral vestibulospinal tract
15. Ventral corticospinal tract
16. Central canal
18. Dorsal spinocerebellar tract
19. Ventral spinocerebellar tract
20. Dorsal intermediate sulcus
21. Accessory nucleus (XI)
23. Cuneate fasciculus
24. Lateral spinothalamic and spinotectal tracts
25. Rubrospinal tract

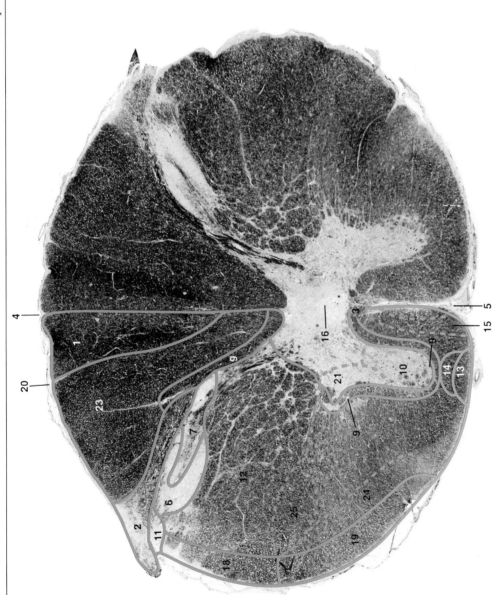

FIGURE 6-9.
Transverse section through the upper cervical spinal cord (C1).

Atlas of the Human Brain, by Lothar Jennes,
Harold H. Traurig, and P. Michael Conn.
J. B. Lippincott Company, Philadelphia, © 1995.

The Vasculature of the Brain

c h a p t e r 7

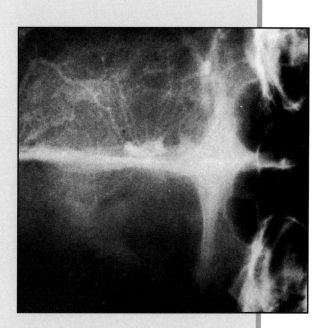

Chapter 7

IMAGING THE CENTRAL NERVOUS SYSTEM IN THE LIVING PATIENT

Several imaging methods are commonly employed to visualize the morphology and vasculature of the central nervous system, to facilitate analysis of pathologic alterations, and to assess the outcomes of head trauma. Full descriptions of the technical aspects of these imaging methods and detailed interpretations of the resulting images are beyond the scope of this atlas; the list of Selected Readings suggests several more complete sources. This chapter will discuss the most common imaging methods.

Angiography is the oldest specialized imaging technique. It requires rapid intravascular injection of an x-ray-opaque "contrast" medium (water soluble organic iodide compound) into either a vertebral or carotid artery. In the normal brain, the contrast medium does not pass the blood–brain barrier and therefore remains in the vascular space. Central nervous system vasculature is visualized through a series of x-ray images of the head in the lateral or anterior-posterior plane made at very short time intervals following the contrast medium injection. Blood carrying the contrast medium is visualized first in the major branches of the vertebral or internal carotid artery, and subsequently in the arterioles, capillary beds, veins, and dural sinuses.

Normal vascular patterns are fairly constant; deviations from the normal patterns suggest the presence of intracranial lesions that diminish blood flow or shift the position of vessels. Angiography permits visualization of vascular stenosis, occlusions, malformations and aneurysms; displacement of vessels suggests a "space-occupying" lesion such as a tumor. Although neural structures are not imaged with this technique, their known anatomical relationships to the vasculature permits their localization.

Computed tomography (CT-scan) was introduced to clinical practice in the 1970s. It provides images that are computer reconstructions of head and brain tissue x-ray densities. These images are produced by passing a series of collimated x-ray beams through the head in a horizontal plane from several points around the circumference of the head. The differential densities of structures encountered by

each collimated x-ray beam as it passes through the head causes a decrement in x-ray energy. These minute differences are detected by sensors and conveyed to a computer. The data are collated and the densities of components in the head and brain at any point in that horizontal plane are calculated. The results are displayed as a computer-constructed horizontal "slice" through the head. A series of horizontal slices are produced at 5 to 10 mm intervals. The thickness of the slice and the plane of section can be varied for special purposes, and contrast media may be introduced into the vasculature or ventricles to enhance their visualization.

Magnetic resonance imaging (MRI) is a noninvasive technique that produces images similar to CT-scans, but MRI provides images of superior resolution, is more versatile, and, most importantly, relies on magnetic energy rather than X-rays.

The term magnetic resonance derives from the observation that atomic nuclei with odd numbers of protons or neutrons respond like magnets and align parallel with respect to the axis of an externally-applied magnetic field. In clinically useful MRI devices, the strength of the external magnetic fields is about 20 kilogauss or 2.0 Tesla and is generated by a superconducting magnet. Once aligned with respect to the external magnetic field, each species of atomic nuclei (or element) will emit a characteristic pattern of magnetic resonance energy following the application of a sequence of radiofrequency pulses which perturbs their alignment. (The pulse frequency is also referred to as repetition time or TR). The times required for buildup of emitted magnetic resonance energy and subsequent return to equilibrium following the sequence of radiofrequency energy pulses are physical characteristics of each element and are referred to as T1 and T2 intervals respectively. (The time between application of TR and detection of signal is the echo time or TE.)

Water, cerebrospinal fluid, and dilute liquids have long T1 intervals, whereas water bound to macromolecules, bone and blood, has short T1 intervals. "Solid" tissue components have short T2 times, whereas T2 for dilute solutions are long. By taking advantage of these characteristic atomic and molecular behaviors in magnetic fields, and by altering the external magnetic field strength and pulse sequence (TR), the resulting MR image will appear quite different, that is, will emphasize certain components of the tissue while others are less well-resolved.

Sensing and collating the resonance frequencies provides data for computer construction of a map representing the concentration of a particular element in the head and brain. Images are represented as "slices" and can be generated in any plane. Body tissues, including the brain, are composed largely of water. Further, the hydrogen atoms in water provide strong resonance signals; thus, MR images are computer-constructed maps of hydrogen atom concentrations in tissues. MR provides high resolution images of gray and white matter components because of their differences in water content and the degree to which the water is "bound" to macromolecules. Moreover, the differences in water binding or mobility and content in tumors, bone, blood (hemorrhages), and tissue altered through disease, ischemia, or trauma also produce characteristic images.

MRI techniques can be varied to facilitate special diagnostic purposes. Agents that alter the magnetic characteristics during MR imaging provide image enhancement. Thus, the same structure or space may image white (intense) or black (void). Gadolinium, a rare earth element, when incorporated into a gadopentetate dimeglumine (Gd-DTPA) mol-

ecule is an injectable MR contrast-enhancing substance in common use; others are colloidal suspensions or iron EDTA or magnesium EDTA.

Common settings during MRI employ long TR combined with short TE times. This weights the imaging in favor of T1 characteristics—bone and cerebrospinal fluid are dark (devoid of signal), while fat (in the dermis of the scalp or orbital fat) is white (intense signal). However, if long TR time is combined with long TE time, the imaging is weighted in favor of T2 characteristics—cerebrospinal fluid and fat are white, bone and *flowing* blood are dark. It should be noted that in the usual MR image, bone is devoid of signal and therefore does not image; this is in contrast to the intense imaging of bone in CT scans. (However, often it may appear as if bone is imaging in MR due to the fat content of the marrow.) On the other hand, fat is brightly imaged in MRI, but not in CT scans.

Selected Readings

Fischer HW, Ketonen L. Radiographic neuroanatomy: A working atlas. New York: McGraw-Hill, 1991. (ISBN) 0-07-021101-9)

Grossman CB. Magnetic resonance imaging and computed tomography of the head and spine. Baltimore: Williams & Wilkins, 1990. (ISBN 0-683-03768-4)

1. Anterior cerebral artery
2. Frontopolar artery
3. Pericallosal artery
4. Callosomarginal artery
5. Parietaloccipital artery
6. Calcarine artery

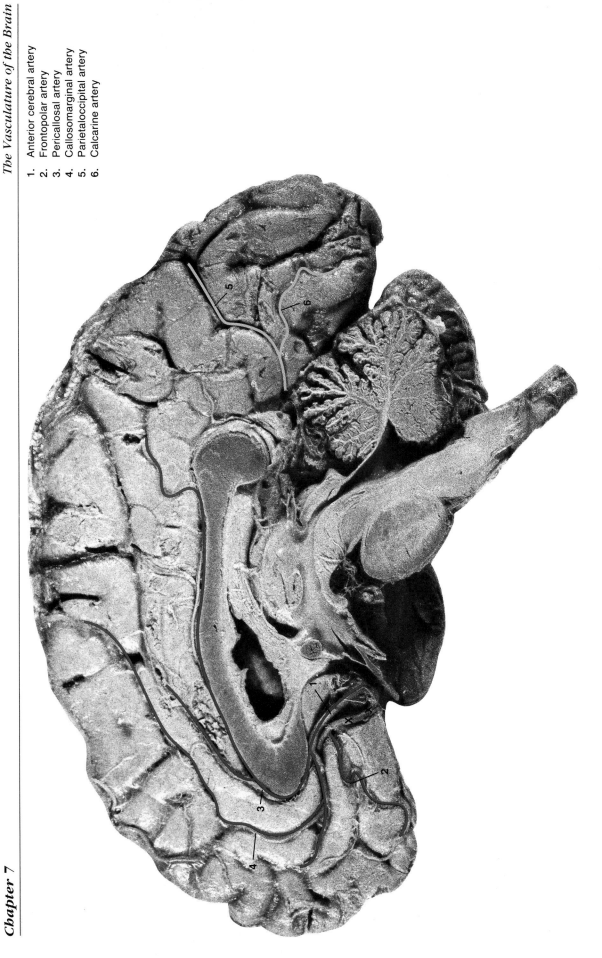

FIGURE 7-1.

Main arterial branches originating from the anterior cerebral artery (*red*) and from the posterior cerebral artery (*pink*) seen on a midsaggital section of the brain. In this specimen, the anterior cerebral artery bifurcates more proximal than usual (xx).

Chapter 7

1. Great vein of Galen
2. Internal cerebral vein
3. Inferior sagittal sinus
4. Straight sinus
5. Thalamus
6. Interventricular foramen of Monro
7. Splenium of corpus callosum

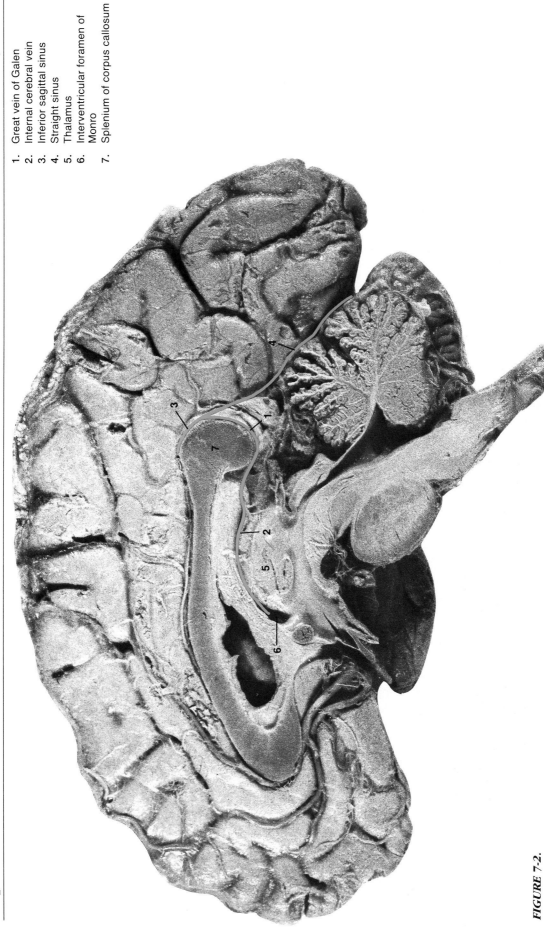

FIGURE 7-2.

Major veins draining into the straight sinus seen on a midsagittal section of the brain. The venous drainage of structures lying deep in the cerebral hemisphere collect on the surface of the lateral ventricles and combine at the interventricular foramen of Monro (*6*) to form the paired internal cerebral veins (*2*). These course posteriorly in the roof of the third ventricle and unite in the region of the pineal to form the great cerebral vein of Galen (*1*). A number of venous structures, including the inferior sagittal sinus (*3*), basal vein, and the superior cerebellar veins (not shown) join to form the straight sinus (*4*). The venous blood follows the straight sinus posteriorly and enters the confluence. (Compare with Figure 7-6.)

The Vasculature of the Brain

1. Internal carotid artery
2. Carotid siphon (intracavernous segment of internal carotid artery)
3. Middle cerebral artery, temporoparietal branch
4. Branches of middle cerebral artery
5. Anterior cerebral artery
6. Pericallosal artery
7. Ophthalmic artery
8. Orbitofrontal artery
9. Callosomarginal artery

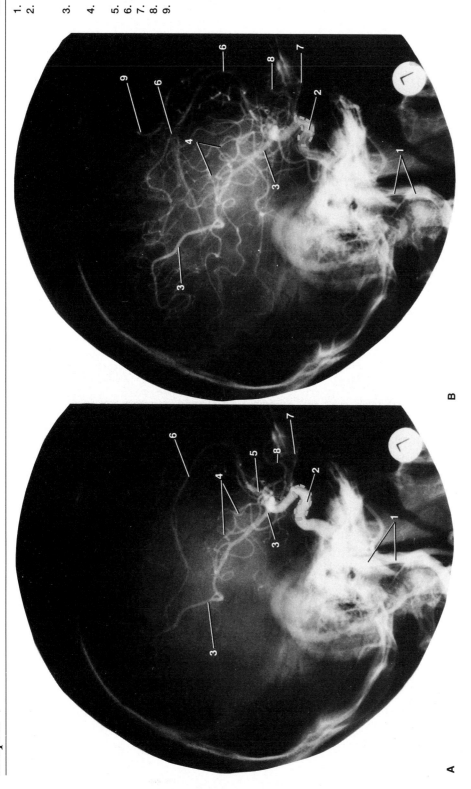

A

B

FIGURE 7-3.

Series of lateral view angiograms taken at consecutive intervals after injection of a contrast medium into the carotid system. At the earliest stage (**A**), only the major arterial branches of the internal carotid artery are visible. (**B**) The contrast medium has reached the smaller arteries. (**C**) The capillary phase is seen. (**D**) The early venous phase is shown. (**E**) The mid-venous phase. (**F**) The late venous phase.

Chapter 7

2. Carotid siphon
   (intracavernous segment of
   internal carotid artery)
3. Middle cerebral artery,
   temporoparietal branch
7. Ophthalmic artery
10. Middle cerebral vein
11. Greater anastomotic vein of
    Trolard
12. Lesser anastomotic vein of
    Labbe

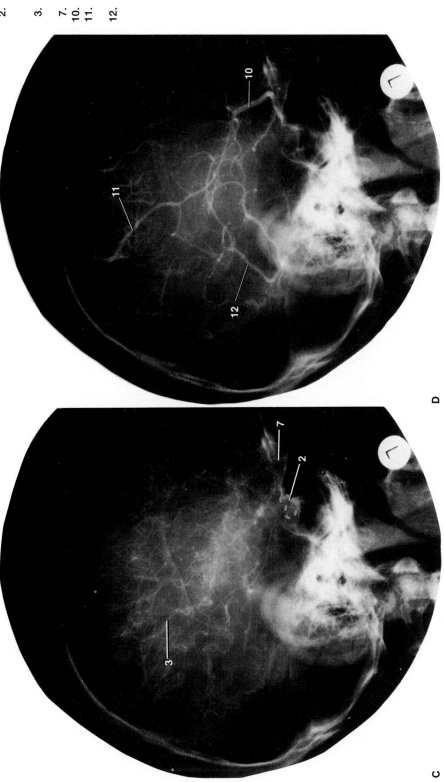

FIGURE 7-3 *Continued*

The Vasculature of the Brain

10. Middle cerebral vein
11. Greater anastomotic vein of Trolard
12. Lesser anastomotic vein of Labbe
13. Superior sagittal sinus
14. Confluence of sinuses
15. Transverse sinus
16. Inferior sagittal sinus
17. Thalamostriate vein
18. Venous angle (intraventricular foramen of Monro)
19. Internal cerebral vein
20. Great cerebral vein of Galen
21. Straight sinus

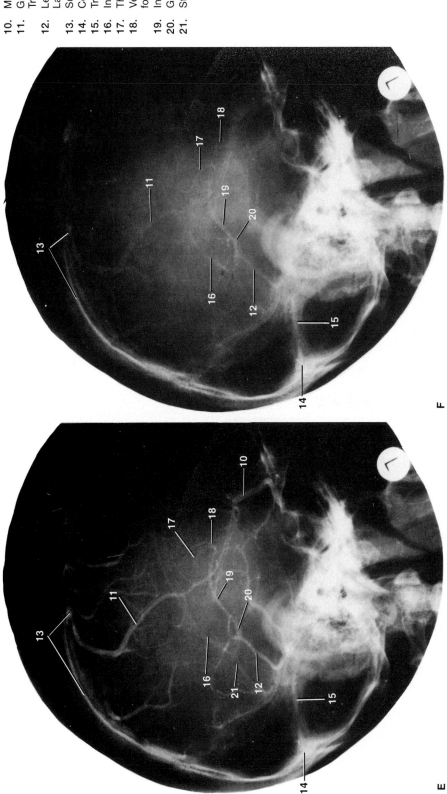

FIGURE 7-3 Continued

The Vasculature of the Brain

1. Internal carotid artery
2. Carotid siphon (intracavernous segment of internal carotid artery)
5. Anterior cerebral artery
22. Middle cerebral artery (M-1 segment)
23. Branches of middle cerebral artery on surface of insula
24. Branches of anterior cerebral artery

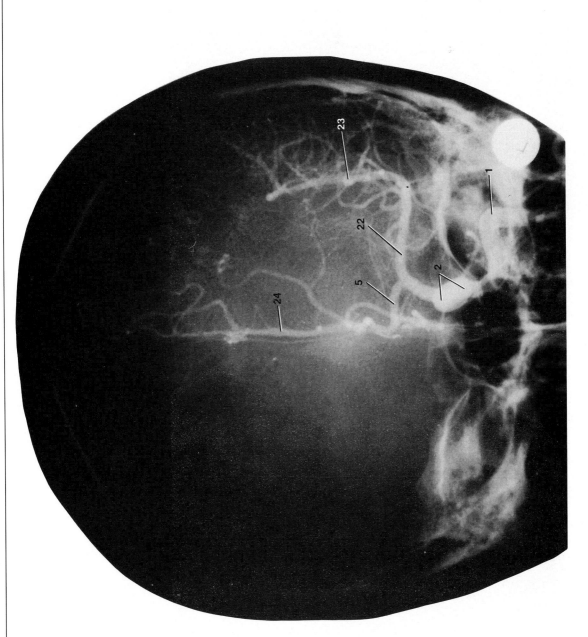

FIGURE 7-4.

Angiogram after injection of a contrast medium into the carotid system during the arterial phase. Anterior–posterior view.

The Vasculature of the Brain

25. Vertebral artery
26. Basilar artery
27. Posterior cerebral artery
28. Posterior cerebral artery, parieto-occipital branch
29. Superior cerebellar artery

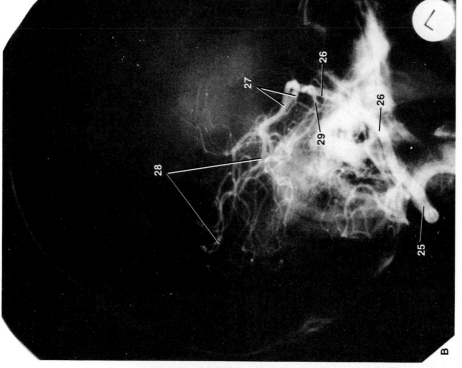

FIGURE 7-5.
Angiograms after injection of a contast medium into the vertebral artery during the arterial phase.
(**A**) Anterior–posterior view. (**B**) Lateral view.

The Vasculature of the Brain

13. Superior sagittal sinus
14. Confluence of sinuses
15. Transverse sinus
19. Internal cerebral vein
20. Great cerebral vein of Galen
21. Straight sinus
30. Cerebral hemispheric branches, bridging vein
31. Occipital sinus
32. Basal vein of Rosenthal
33. Superior cerebellar vein

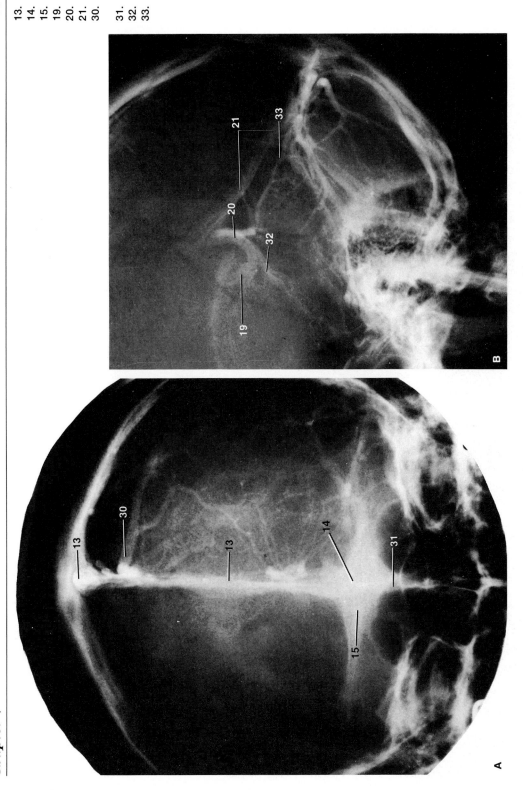

FIGURE 7-6.

Angiograms after injection of a contrast medium showing the venous phase. (**A**) Anterior–posterior view. (**B**) Lateral view.

25. Vertebral artery
26. Basilar artery
27. Posterior cerebral artery
29. Superior cerebellar artery
34. Aneurysm at summit of basilar
    artery

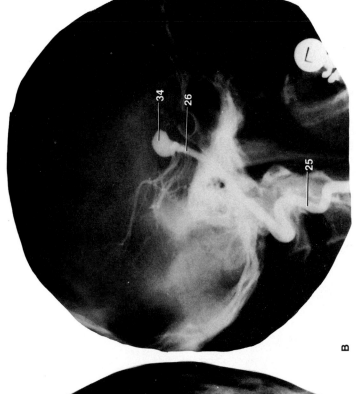

A

B

FIGURE 7-7.

Angiograms after injection of a contrast medium into the vertebral artery during the arterial phase
showing an aneurysm of the summit of the basilar artery. The aneurysm lies in the interpeduncular
cistern. (**A**) Anterior–posterior view. (**B**) Lateral view.

1. Internal carotid artery
5. Anterior cerebral artery
22. Middle cerebral artery
23. Branches of middle cerebral artery on surface of insula
25. Vertebral artery
26. Basilar artery
27. Posterior cerebral artery
28. Posterior cerebral artery, parieto-occipital branch
35. Aneurysm

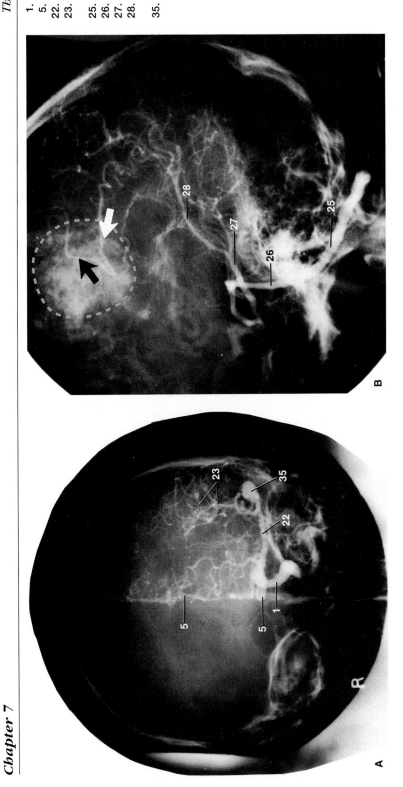

FIGURE 7-8.

Angiograms after injection of a contrast medium into the carotid system and into the vertebral artery showing an aneurysm of the middle cerebral artery and the capillary network associated with a tumor (B, *dotted area*). The aneurysm lies in the lateral fissure, while the tumor is located in the parietal lobe. The tumor has evoked the formation of abnormal blood vessels supplying that area (B, *arrows*).
(A) Anterior–posterior view; **(B)** Lateral view.

Atlas of the Human Brain, by Lothar Jennes,
Harold H. Traurig, and P. Michael Conn.
J. B. Lippincott Company, Philadelphia. © 1995.

Computed Tomography (CT) and Magnetic Resonance Imaging (MRI) of the Brain and Spinal Cord

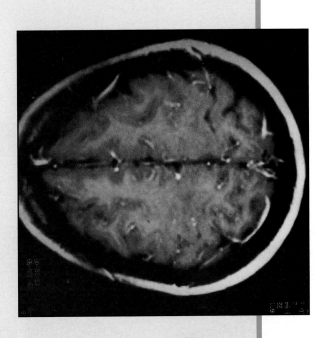

8

c h a p t e r

Computed Tomography (CT) and Magnetic Resonance Imaging (MRI) of the Brain and Spinal Cord

1. Anterior falx
2. Posterior falx
3. Parietal bone
4. White matter of cerebral hemispheres (centrum semiovale)
5. Gray matter of cerebral hemispheres

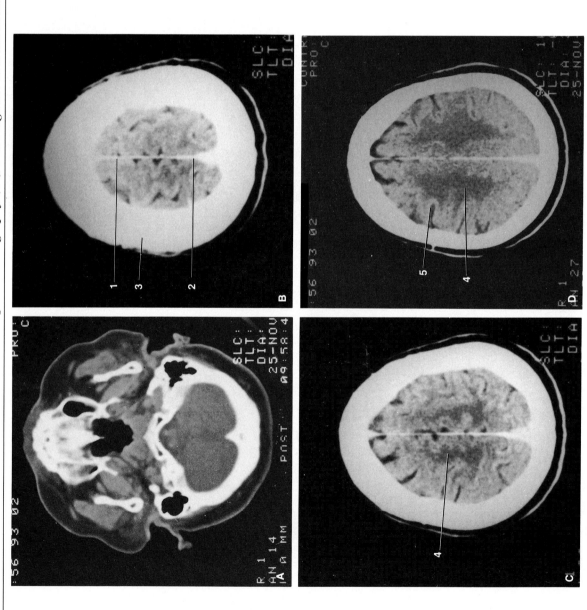

FIGURE 8-1.

(A–L) Series of computed tomographic images taken in a horizontal plane (superior to inferior) through the head of a normal subject. The images were enhanced to reveal certain aspects of the vasculature. **A** serves for orientation purposes.

Computed Tomography (CT) and Magnetic Resonance Imaging (MRI) of the Brain and Spinal Cord

1. Anterior falx
2. Posterior falx
6. Body of the lateral ventricle
7. Anterior horn of the lateral ventricle
8. Posterior horn of the lateral ventricle
9. Septum pellucidum
10. Fornix
11. Head of caudate nucleus
12. Internal capsule, anterior limb
13. Lenticular nucleus
14. Interventricular foramen of Monro
15. Internal capsule, posterior limb
16. Thalamus
17. Cavum velum interpositum
18. Internal cerebral vein
19. Choroid plexus in trigone of lateral ventricle
20. Insula cistern
21. Third ventricle
22. Pineal

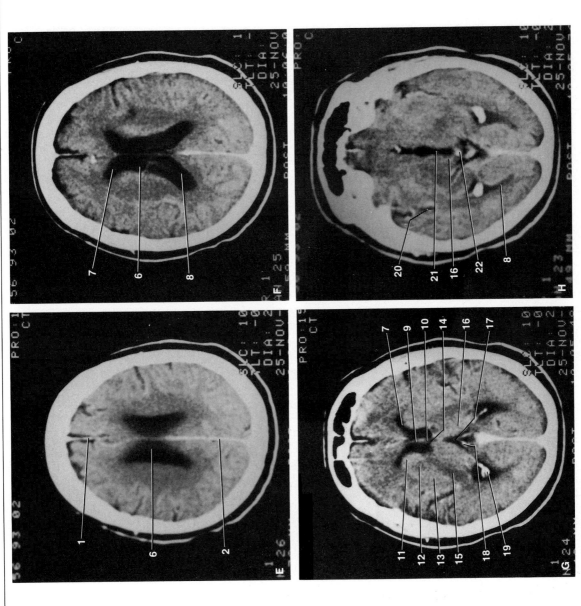

FIGURE 8-1 Continued

Computed Tomography (CT) and Magnetic Resonance Imaging (MRI) of the Brain and Spinal Cord

23. Middle cerebral artery
24. Internal carotid artery
25. Uncus of hippocampus
26. Basilar artery
27. Midbrain
28. Quadrigeminal cistern
29. Vermis of cerebellum
30. Lesser wing of sphenoid bone
31. Anterior clinoid process
32. Temporal lobe
33. Interpeduncular fossa
34. Sella turcica
35. Inferior horn of the lateral ventricle
36. Pons
37. Occipital lobe
38. Fourth ventricle
39. Petrous portion of temporal bone
40. Labyrinth

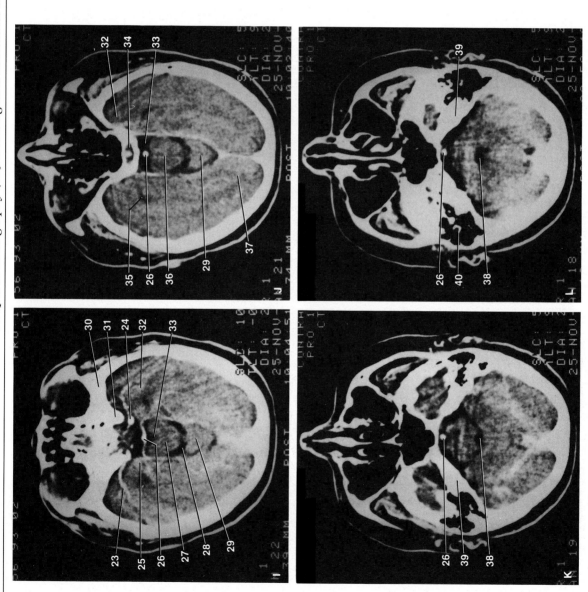

FIGURE 8-1 *Continued*

Computed Tomography (CT) and Magnetic Resonance Imaging (MRI) of the Brain and Spinal Cord

1. Vertebral artery
2. Spinal cord
3. Cisterna magna
4. Medulla
5. Tonsil of cerebellum
6. Cerebellar hemisphere
7. Medullary pyramid
8. Inferior olive nucleus
9. Inferior cerebellar peduncle
10. Fourth ventricle
11. Vermis of cerebellum
12. Medial leminiscus
13. Lateral aperture of Luschka
14. Cerebellar vermis
15. Dentate nucleus

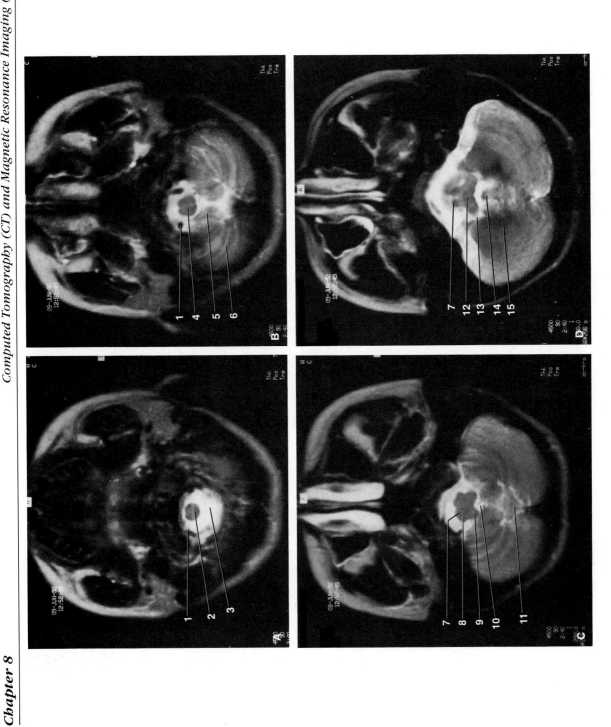

FIGURE 8-2.

(A–L) Series of MR images taken in a horizontal plane (inferior to superior) through the head of a normal subject. The contrast was enhanced to reveal the spaces occupied by cerebrospinal fluid.

Computed Tomography (CT) and Magnetic Resonance Imaging (MRI) of the Brain and Spinal Cord

10. Fourth ventricle
14. Cerebellar vermis
16. Temporal lobe
17. Sphenoid sinus
18. Basilar artery
19. Pontine cistern
20. Middle cerebellar peduncle
21. Straight sinus
22. Internal carotid artery in cavernous sinus
23. Eye
24. Sella turcica
25. Cerebral peduncle
26. Anterior cerebral artery
27. Middle cerebral artery
28. Suprasellar cistern
29. Uncus
30. Posterior cerebral artery
31. Interpeduncular cistern
32. Red nucleus
33. Superior colliculus
34. Quadrigeminal cistern
35. Visual radiations
36. Occipital lobe
37. Posterior horn of lateral ventricle
38. Putamen
39. Insular cistern
40. Third ventricle
41. Thalamus
42. Posterior commissure
43. Trigone of lateral ventricle
44. Transverse gyri of Heschl

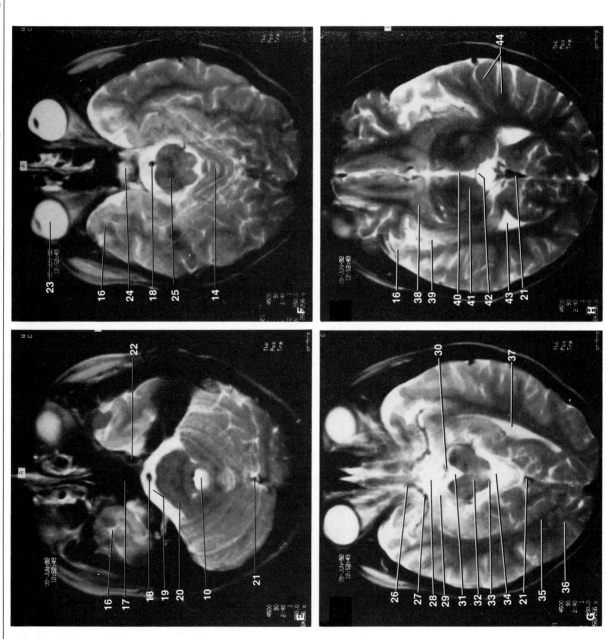

FIGURE 8-2   Continued

Computed Tomography (CT) and Magnetic Resonance Imaging (MRI) of the Brain and Spinal Cord

36. Occipital lobe
37. Posterior horn of lateral ventricle
38. Putamen
41. Thalamus
43. Trigone of lateral ventricle
44. Transverse gyri of Heschl
45. Frontal lobe
46. Interhemispheric fissure
47. Anterior horn of lateral ventricle
48. Head of caudate nucleus
49. Anterior limb of internal capsule
50. Fornix
51. Interventricular foramen of Monro
52. Posterior limb of internal capsule
53. Splenium of corpus callosum
54. Genu of internal capsule
55. External capsule
56. Genu of corpus callosum
57. Septum pellucidum
58. Body of lateral ventricle
59. Insular cortex
60. Centrum semiovale
61. Cortical gray matter
62. Cortical white matter
63. Parietal lobe

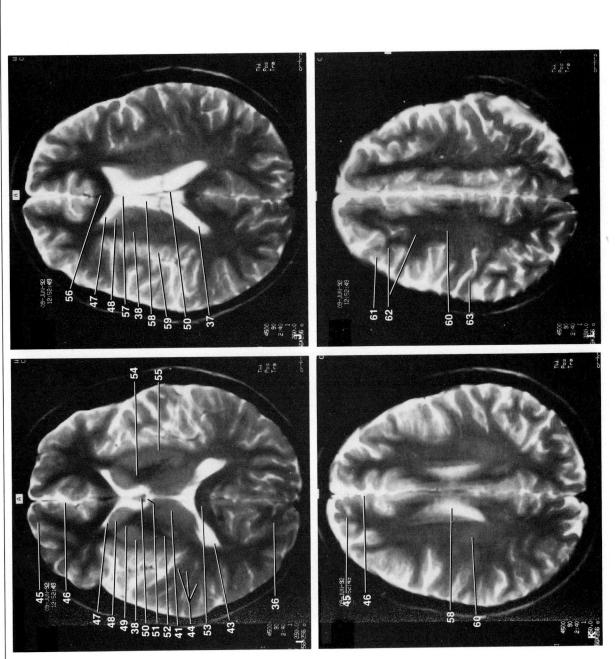

FIGURE 8-2   Continued

Computed Tomography (CT) and Magnetic Resonance Imaging (MRI) of the Brain and Spinal Cord

1. Spinal cord
2. Cisterna magna
3. Caudal medulla
4. Tonsils of the cerebellum
5. Rostral medulla
6. Fourth ventricle
7. Inferior cerebellar peduncle
8. Cerebellar hemispheres
9. Basilar artery
10. Basilar pons
11. Middle cerebellar peduncle

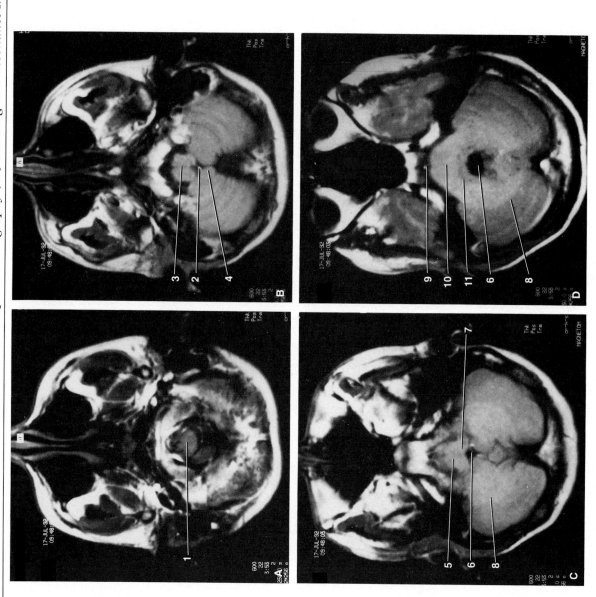

FIGURE 8-3.

(A–L) Series of MR images taken in a horizontal plane (inferior to superior) through the head of a normal subject.

Computed Tomography (CT) and Magnetic Resonance Imaging (MRI) of the Brain and Spinal Cord

6. Fourth ventricle
9. Basilar artery
10. Basilar pons
12. Temporal lobe
13. Tegmentum of pons
14. Optic nerve
15. Cerebral peduncle
16. Red nucleus
17. Cerebral aqueduct
18. Vermis of cerebellum
19. Occipital lobe
20. Uncus of hippocampus
21. Interpeduncular cistern
22. Ambient cistern
23. Quadrigeminal cistern
24. Frontal lobe
25. Interhemispheric fissure
26. Lateral fissure
27. Third ventricle
28. Superior colliculus
29. Head of caudate nucleus
30. Fornix
31. Insula
32. Habenula
33. Posterior horn of the lateral ventricle
34. Visual pathway (geniculo-calcarine tract)
35. Superior sagittal sinus

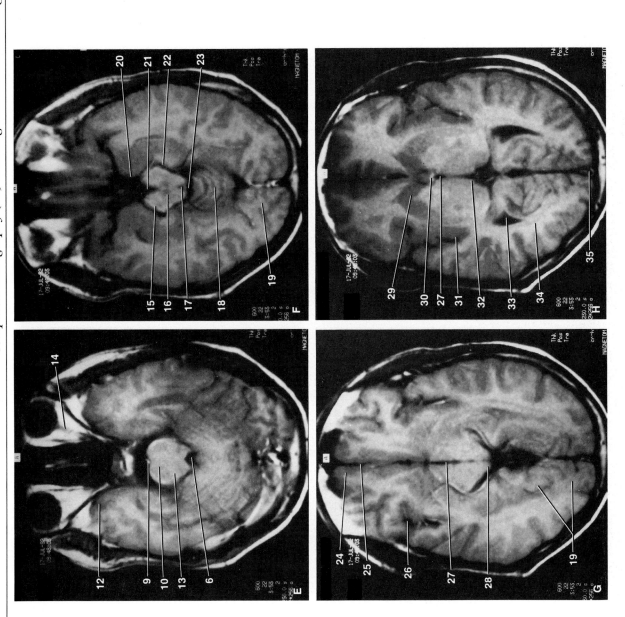

FIGURE 8-3 Continued

103

Computed Tomography (CT) and Magnetic Resonance Imaging (MRI) of the Brain and Spinal Cord

19. Occipital lobe
24. Frontal lobe
29. Head of caudate nucleus
30. Fornix
35. Superior sagittal sinus
36. Genu of the corpus callosum
37. Septum pellucidum
38. Claustrum and external capsule
39. Putamen
40. Internal capsule
41. Thalamus
42. Splenium of the corpus callosum
43. Anterior horn of the lateral ventricle
44. Body of the lateral ventricle
45. Centrum semiovale

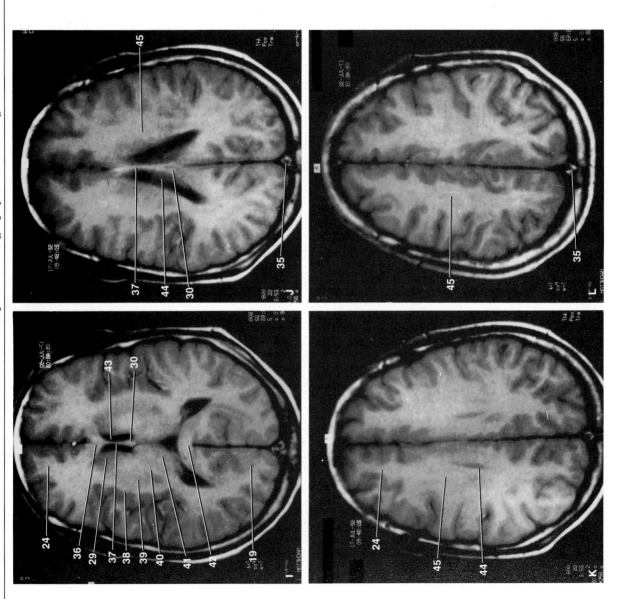

FIGURE 8-3 Continued

Computed Tomography (CT) and Magnetic Resonance Imaging (MRI) of the Brain and Spinal Cord

1. Superior sagittal sinus
2. Interhemispheric cistern
3. Frontal radiations
4. Cortical gray matter
5. Cortical white matter
6. Optic foramen
7. Temporal lobe
8. Frontal lobe
9. Genu of corpus callosum
10. Anterior horn of lateral ventricle
11. Lateral fissure
12. Gyrus rectus
13. Cingulate gyrus
14. Body of corpus callosum
15. Insular cortex

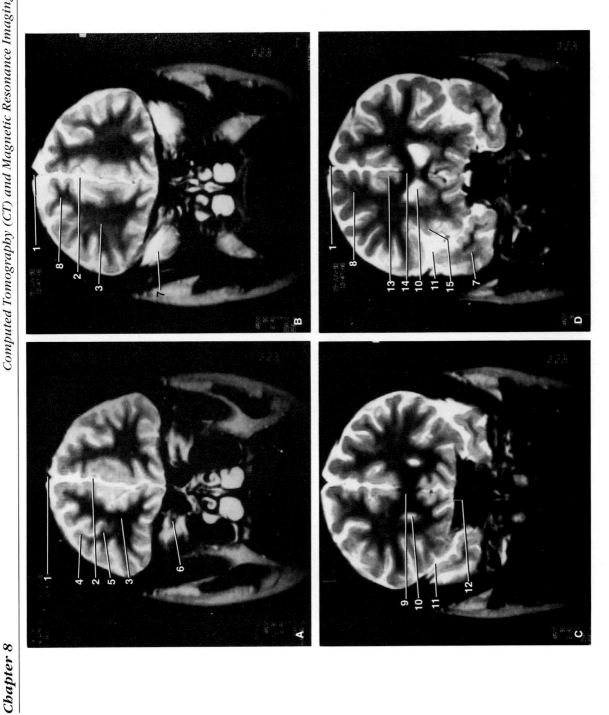

FIGURE 8-4.

(A–L) Series of MR images taken in a coronal plane (anterior to posterior) through the head of a normal subject. The contrast was enhanced to reveal the spaces occupied by cerebrospinal fluid.

Computed Tomography (CT) and Magnetic Resonance Imaging (MRI) of the Brain and Spinal Cord

1. Superior sagittal sinus
7. Temporal lobe
8. Frontal lobe
10. Anterior horn of lateral ventricle
11. Lateral fissure
13. Cingulate gyrus
14. Body of corpus callosum
15. Insular cortex
16. Head of caudate nucleus
17. Septum pellucidum
18. Anterior limb of internal capsule
19. Putamen
20. Anterior cerebral artery
21. Internal carotid artery
22. Corona radiata
23. Septum (parolfactory gyrus)
24. Middle cerebral artery
25. Amygdala
26. Uncus
27. Fornix
28. Interventricular foramen of Monro
29. Basilar artery
30. Posterior cerebral artery
31. Middle cerebral artery, Sylvian branch
32. Third ventricle
33. Hypothalamus
34. Interpeduncular cistern
35. Basilar pons
60. Massa intermedia

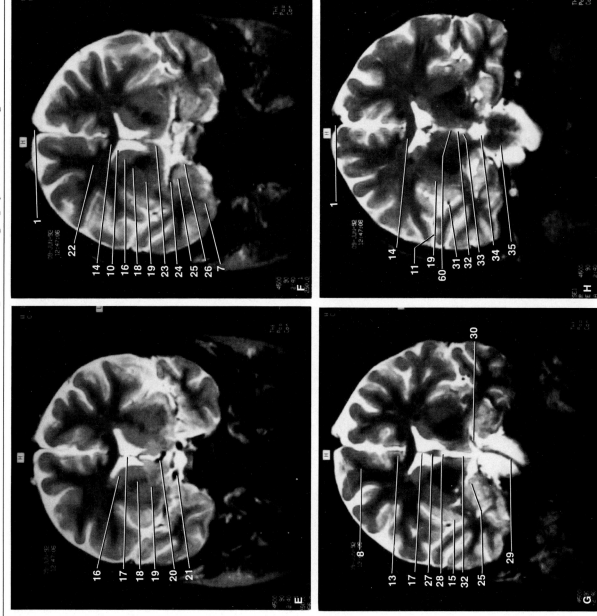

FIGURE 8-4   Continued

1. Superior sagittal sinus
8. Frontal lobe
10. Anterior horn of lateral ventricle
13. Cingulate gyrus
14. Body of corpus callosum
15. Insular cortex
16. Head of caudate nucleus
27. Fornix
32. Third ventricle
35. Basilar pons
36. Internal cerebral vein
37. Thalamus
38. Red nucleus
39. Substantia nigra
40. Posterior limb of internal capsule
41. Cerebral peduncle
42. Hippocampus
43. Inferior horn of lateral ventricle
44. Middle cerebellar peduncle
45. Olivary nucleus (medulla)
46. Body of lateral ventricle
47. Quadrigeminal cistern
48. Superior colliculus
49. Inferior colliculus
50. Cerebral aqueduct
51. Superior cerebellar peduncle
52. Fourth ventricle
53. Medulla
54. Splenium of corpus callosum
55. Trigone of lateral ventricle
56. Vermis of cerebellum
57. Cisterna magna
58. Cerebellar hemisphere
59. Occipital lobe

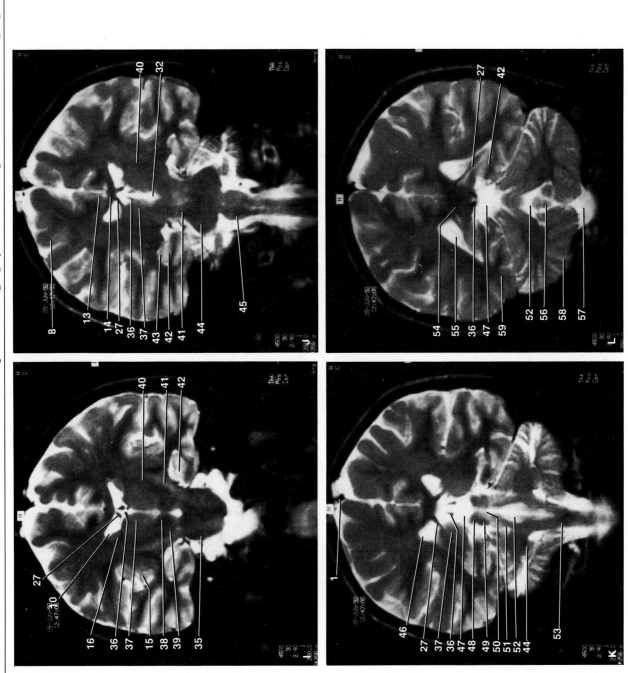

FIGURE 8-4   Continued

Computed Tomography (CT) and Magnetic Resonance Imaging (MRI) of the Brain and Spinal Cord

1. Frontal lobe
2. Lateral fissure
3. Temporal lobe
4. Parietal lobe
5. Occipital lobe
6. Location of the tentorium cerebelli
7. Cerebellum
8. Transverse sinus
9. Insular cortex
10. Corona radiata
11. Trigone of lateral ventricle
12. Hippocampus
13. Temporal pole

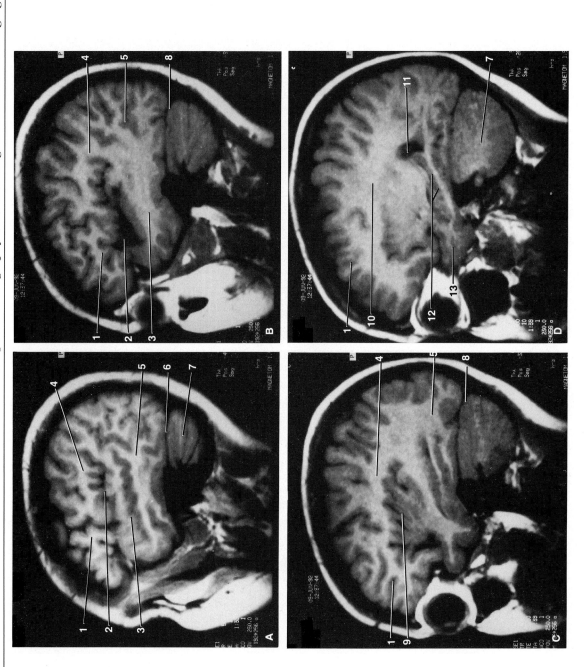

FIGURE 8-5.

(A–L) Series of MR images taken in a sagittal plane (lateral to medial) through the head of a normal subject.

Computed Tomography (CT) and Magnetic Resonance Imaging (MRI) of the Brain and Spinal Cord

7. Cerebellum
8. Transverse sinus
13. Temporal pole
14. Lenticular nucleus
15. Body of corpus callosum
16. Anterior horn of lateral ventricle
17. Head of caudate nucleus
18. Parieto-occipital fissure
19. Fornix
20. Thalamus
21. Splenium of corpus callosum
22. Calcarine fissure
23. Quadrigeminal cistern
24. Basilar pons
25. Middle cerebellar peduncle
26. Tonsils of cerebellum
27. Internal cerebral vein
28. Anterior cerebral artery
29. Optic chiasm
30. Medulla
31. Superior colliculus
32. Inferior colliculus
33. Superior cerebellar peduncle
34. Fourth ventricle
35. Body of lateral ventricle
36. Genu of corpus callosum
37. Interventricular foramen of Monro
38. Anterior commissure
39. Septum
40. Lamina terminalis
41. Hypothalamus
42. Optic nerve
43. Mammillary body
44. Interpeduncular cistern
45. Paracentral lobule
46. Cingulate gyrus
47. Posterior commissure
48. Tectum of midbrain
49. Cerebral aqueduct

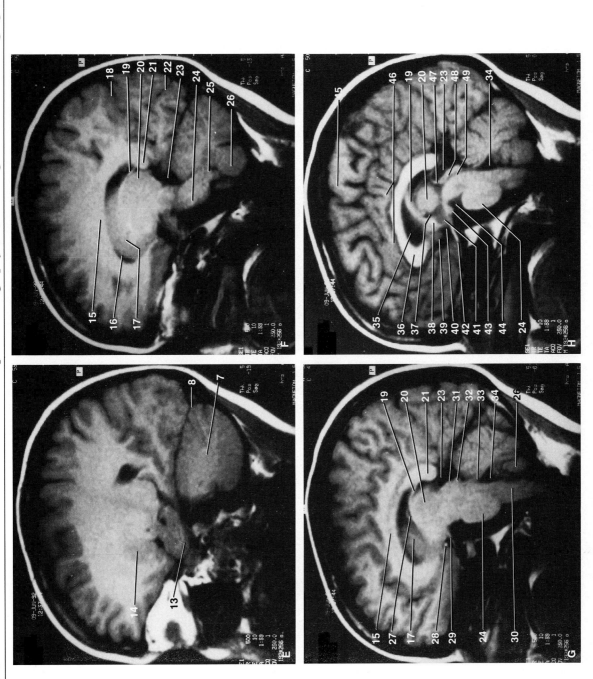

FIGURE 8-5 *Continued*

Chapter 8

Computed Tomography (CT) and Magnetic Resonance Imaging (MRI) of the Brain and Spinal Cord

1. Frontal lobe
4. Parietal lobe
5. Occipital lobe
7. Cerebellum
9. Insular cortex
10. Corona radiata
11. Trigone of lateral ventricle
12. Hippocampus
13. Temporal pole
15. Body of corpus callosum
17. Head of caudate nucleus
19. Fornix
20. Thalamus
21. Splenium of corpus callosum
23. Quadrigeminal cistern
35. Body of lateral ventricle
39. Septum (parolfactory gyrus)
42. Optic nerve
44. Interpeduncular cistern
46. Cingulate gyrus
50. Posterior horn of lateral ventricle

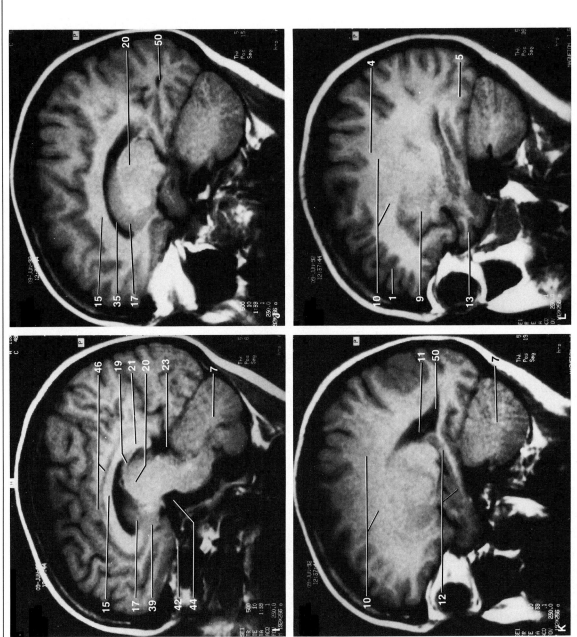

FIGURE 8-5 Continued

Computed Tomography (CT) and Magnetic Resonance Imaging (MRI) of the Brain and Spinal Cord

1. Temporal lobe
2. Cortical gray matter
3. Cortical white matter
4. Frontal lobe
5. Parietal lobe
6. Location of the tentorium cerebelli
7. Hemisphere of cerebellum
8. Lateral fissure

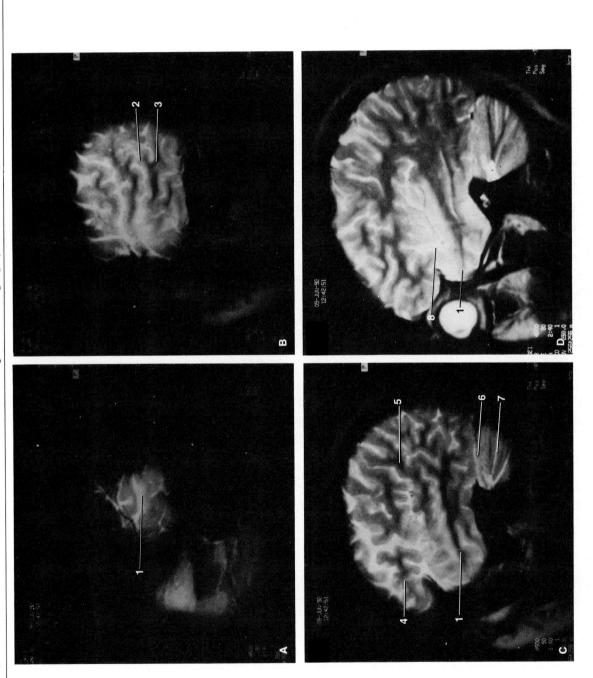

FIGURE 8-6.

(**A–L**) Series of MR images taken in a sagittal plane (lateral to medial) through the head of a normal subject. The contrast was enhanced to reveal the spaces occupied by cerebrospinal fluid.

Chapter 8

Computed Tomography (CT) and Magnetic Resonance Imaging (MRI) of the Brain and Spinal Cord

4. Frontal lobe
7. Hemisphere of cerebellum
9. Insular cortex
10. Middle cerebral artery
11. Eye
12. Amygdala
13. Trigone of lateral ventricle
14. Posterior horn of lateral ventricle
15. Hippocampus
16. Head of caudate nucleus
17. Middle cerebral artery
18. Vertebral artery
19. Thalamus
20. Body of corpus callosum
21. Anterior horn of lateral ventricle
22. Genu of corpus callosum
23. Anterior cerebral artery
24. Basilar pons
25. Inferior olive nucleus
26. Fornix
27. Splenium of corpus callosum
28. Calcarine fissure
29. Superior colliculus
30. Fourth ventricle
31. Tonsil of cerebellum
32. Cisterna magna
33. Cingulate gyrus
34. Body of lateral ventricle
35. Pericallosal artery
36. Anterior commissure
37. Septum
38. Hypothalamus
39. Mammillary body
40. Interpeduncular cistern
41. Basilar artery
42. Pineal
43. Quadrigeminal cistern
44. Tectum of mesencephalon
45. Cerebral aqueduct
46. Anterior medullary velum
47. Medulla
51. Cerebellar white matter and deep cerebellar nuclei
52. Vermis of cerebellum
53. Periorbital adipose tissue

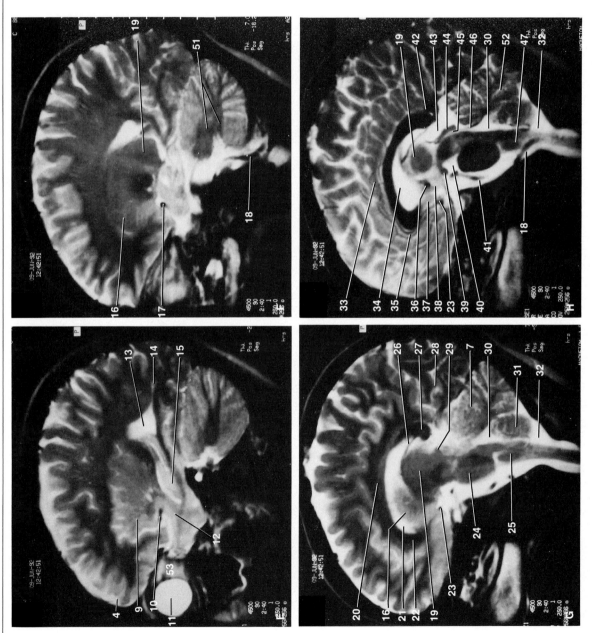

FIGURE 8-6   Continued

112

Computed Tomography (CT) and Magnetic Resonance Imaging (MRI) of the Brain and Spinal Cord

1. Temporal lobe
4. Frontal lobe
6. Location of the tentorium cerebelli
9. Insular cortex
10. Middle cerebral artery
11. Eye
13. Trigone of lateral ventricle
14. Posterior horn of lateral ventricle
15. Hippocampus
16. Head of caudate nucleus
20. Body of corpus callosum
21. Anterior horn of lateral ventricle
22. Genu of corpus callosum
26. Fornix
27. Splenium of corpus callosum
29. Superior colliculus
37. Septum (parolfactory gyrus)
48. Posterior cerebral artery
49. Inferior colliculus
50. Occipital lobe
51. Cerebellar white matter and deep cerebellar nuclei
53. Periorbital adipose tissue

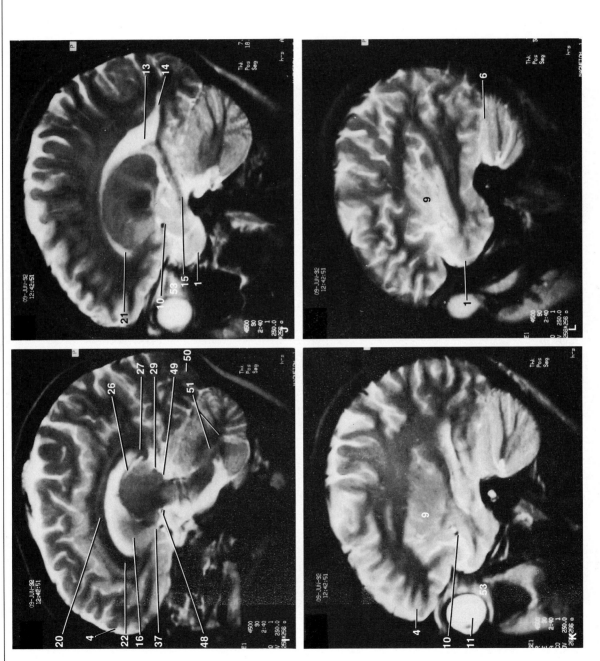

FIGURE 8-6 Continued

Computed Tomography (CT) and Magnetic Resonance Imaging (MRI) of the Brain and Spinal Cord

1. Superior sagittal sinus
2. Frontal lobe
3. Interhemispheric fissure
4. Centrum semiovale
5. Parietal lobe
6. Occipital lobe
7. Head of caudate nucleus
8. Anterior horn of lateral ventricle
9. Septum pellucidum
10. Internal cerebral vein
11. Insular cortex
12. Splenium of corpus callosum
13. Glomus of choroid plexus in trigone
14. Trigone of lateral ventricle
15. Great cerebral vein of Galen
16. Cingulate gyrus
17. Fornix
18. Third ventricle
19. Thalamus
20. Straight sinus
21. Globus pallidus
22. Putamen
23. Anterior commissure
24. Massa intermedia
25. Lateral fissure
26. Posterior horn of lateral ventricle
27. Posterior cerebral artery
28. Superior colliculus
29. Middle cerebral artery, Sylvian branch
30. Temporal lobe

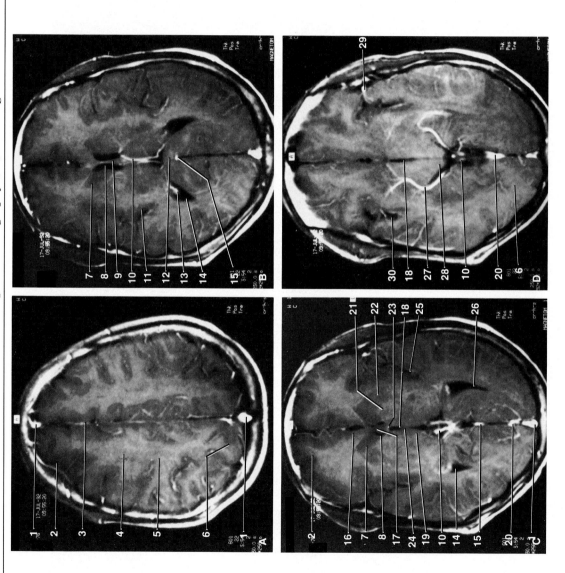

FIGURE 8-7.

(A–L) Comparison of two series of MRIs taken at different enhancement settings in a horizontal plane (superior to inferior) through the head of a normal subject. **A** through **F** are enhanced to reveal blood vessels; **G** through **L** are not enhanced.

Computed Tomography (CT) and Magnetic Resonance Imaging (MRI) of the Brain and Spinal Cord

2. Frontal lobe
3. Interhemispheric fissure
5. Parietal lobe
7. Head of caudate nucleus
12. Splenium of corpus callosum
14. Trigone of lateral ventricle
19. Thalamus
22. Putamen
28. Superior colliculus
29. Middle cerebral artery, Sylvian branch
30. Temporal lobe
31. Uncus
32. Interpeduncular cistern
33. Ambient cistern
34. Quadrigeminal cistern
35. Vermis of cerebellum
36. Confluence of sinuses
37. Amygdala
38. Hippocampus
39. Inferior horn of lateral ventricle
40. Eye
41. Periorbital fat tissue
42. Nasal cavity
43. Basilar artery
44. Internal carotid artery
45. Pons
46. Flocculus of cerebellum
47. Fourth ventricle
48. Sigmoid sinus
49. Cerebellar hemisphere
50. Transverse sinus
51. Superior petrosal sinus
52. Callosomarginal artery
53. Cingulate gyrus
54. Pericallosal artery
55. Cortical gray matter
56. Cortical white matter
57. Body of lateral ventricle
58. Corona radiata
59. Anterior cerebral artery
60. Genu of corpus callosum
61. Anterior limb of internal capsule

continued

115

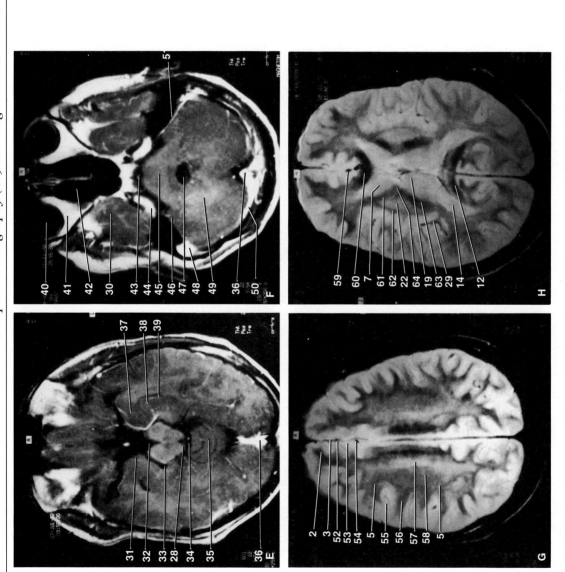

FIGURE 8-7   *Continued*

Computed Tomography (CT) and Magnetic Resonance Imaging (MRI) of the Brain and Spinal Cord

62. External capsule (with claustrum)
63. Posterior limb of internal capsule
64. Genu of internal capsule

2. Frontal lobe
5. Parietal lobe
8. Anterior horn of lateral ventricle
10. Internal cerebral vein
11. Insular cortex
19. Thalamus
27. Posterior cerebral artery
28. Superior colliculus
29. Middle cerebral artery, Sylvian branch
30. Temporal lobe
35. Vermis of cerebellum
40. Eye
43. Basilar artery
49. Cerebellar hemisphere
59. Anterior cerebral artery
62. External capsule (with claustrum)
65. Mammillothalamic tract
66. Pineal
67. Visual radiations
68. Frontal pole
69. Postcommissural fornix
70. Insular cistern
71. Cerebral peduncle
72. Substantia nigra
73. Red nucleus
74. Lateral fissure
75. Middle cerebral artery
76. Pons

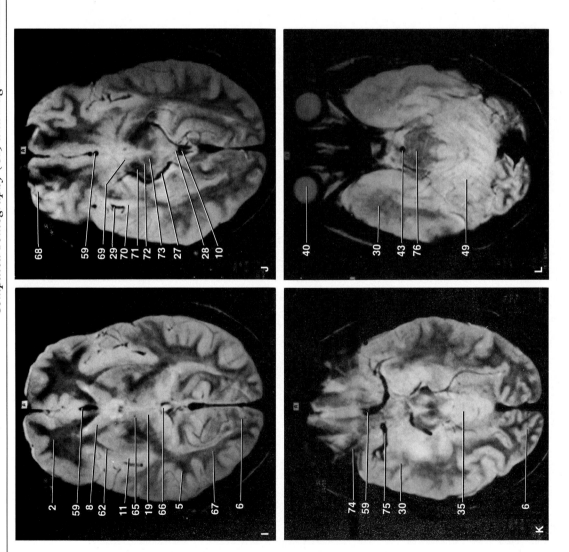

FIGURE 8-7 *Continued*

Computed Tomography (CT) and Magnetic Resonance Imaging (MRI) of the Brain and Spinal Cord

1. Interhemispheric fissure
2. Superior saggital sinus
3. Centrum semiovale
4. Cortical gray matter
5. Cortical white matter

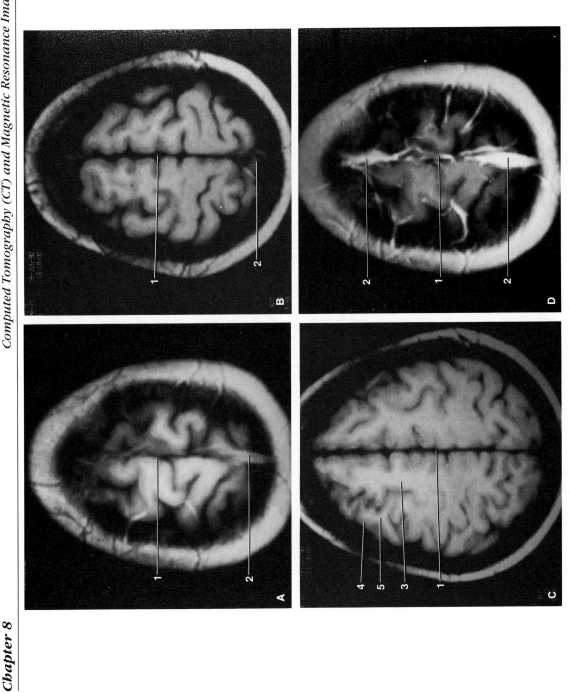

FIGURE 8-8.

(**A–L**) Series of MRIs taken in a horizontal plane through the superior aspects of the cerebrum (superior to inferior) of a normal subject. The characteristics under which the images were obtained were altered to reveal different anatomical relationships; for example, the contrast between gray and white matter is much greater in figures **G**, **H**, and **I** than in **A**, **B**, and **C**. Also, the cerebrospinal fluid images intensely (*white*) in **J** through **L** compared to figures **A** through **C** where the cerebrospinal fluid does not image. **D**, **E**, and **F** reveal some aspects of the vasculature.

1. Interhemispheric fissure
2. Superior saggital sinus
3. Centrum semiovale
4. Cortical gray matter
5. Cortical white matter

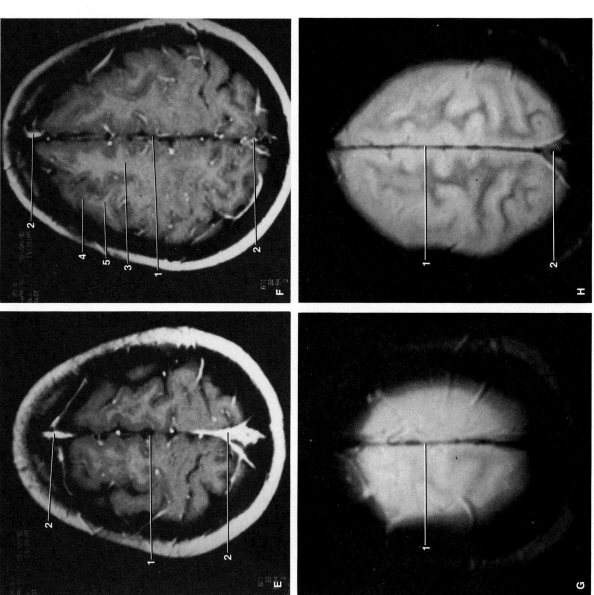

FIGURE 8-8   *Continued*

Computed Tomography (CT) and Magnetic Resonance Imaging (MRI) of the Brain and Spinal Cord

1. Interhemispheric fissure
2. Superior saggital sinus
3. Centrum semiovale
4. Cortical gray matter
5. Cortical white matter

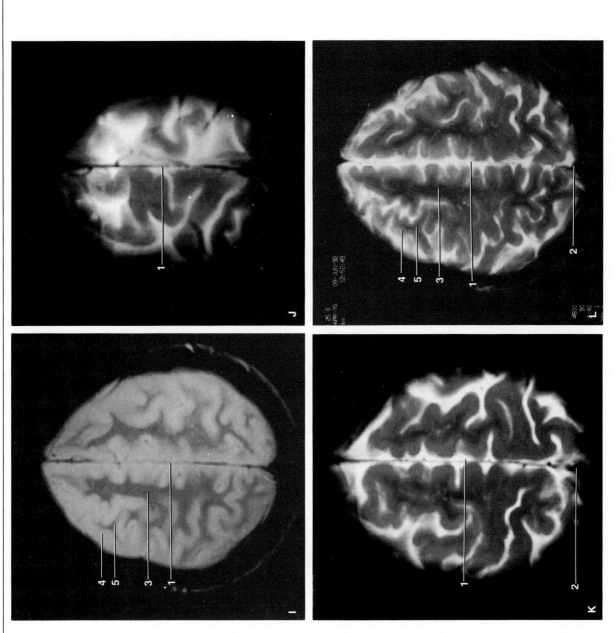

FIGURE 8-8 Continued

Computed Tomography (CT) and Magnetic Resonance Imaging (MRI) of the Brain and Spinal Cord

1. Basilar pons
2. Fourth ventricle
3. Cerebellum
4. Tonsils of cerebellum
5. Obex
6. Cisterna magna
7. Medulla
8. Cervical spinal cord
9. Anterior arch of atlas (C1)
10. Posterior arch of atlas (C1)
11. Dens of axis (C2)
12. Spinous process of axis (C2)
13. Intervertebral disc
14. Conus medullaris
15. Cauda equina
16. Lumbar cistern
17. Caudal end of lumbar cistern
18. Dorsal root ganglion of L3 spinal nerve
19. Dural sleeve, extensions of the dura, arachnoid, subarachnoid, and subdural spaces containing the dorsal and ventral L3 nerve roots in intervertebral foramen
20. Dural sleeve, extensions of the dura, arachnoid, subarachnoid, and subdural spaces containing the dorsal and ventral L4 nerve roots in intervertebral foramen
21. Superior articular process of L5 vertebra
22. Inferior articular process of L5 vertebra
23. Intervertebral foramen

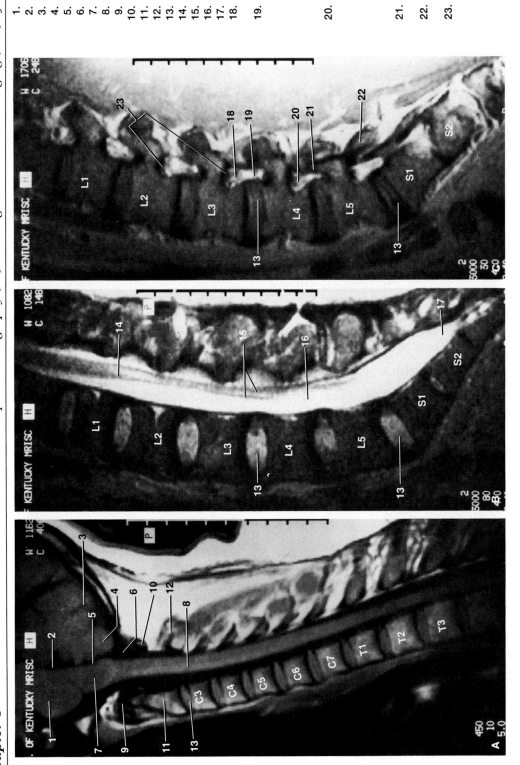

FIGURE 8-9.

MRIs taken in a sagittal (**A**, **B**) and parasagittal (**C**) plane through the brainstem and upper (**A**) and lower (**B**, **C**) spinal cord of a normal individual. The cerebrospinal fluid does not image in **A** but images intensely in figures **B** (*16*) and **C** (*19, 20*).

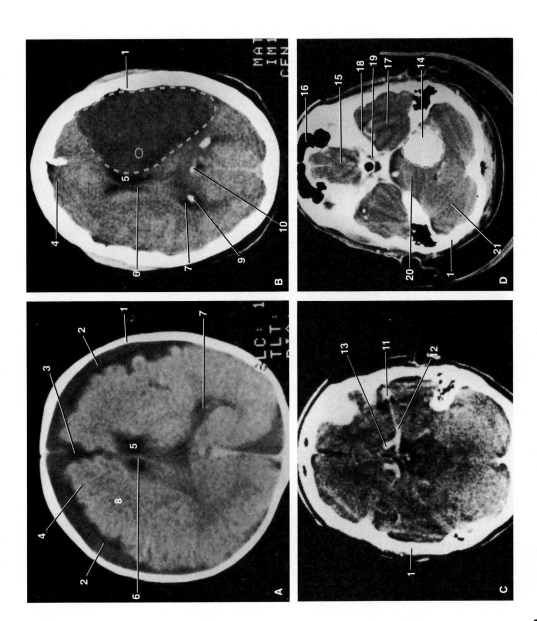

1. Bone tissue of skull
2. Enlarged subdural space
3. Interhemispheric fissure
4. Frontal lobe
5. Anterior horn of lateral ventricle
6. Septum pellucidum
7. Trigone of lateral ventricle
8. Right hemisphere
9. Choroid plexus in the trigone of the lateral ventricle
10. Pineal
11. Aneurysm
12. Middle cerebral artery
13. Internal carotid artery
14. Tumor in posterior cranial fossa
15. Anterior cranial fossa and base of frontal lobe
16. Frontal sinus
17. Middle cranial fossa and base of temporal lobe
18. Lesser wing of sphenoid bone
19. Sella turcica
20. Brainstem
21. Cerebellum

FIGURE 8-10.

CT scans showing examples of pathological conditions. (**A**) CT scan of a patient with bilateral subdural fluid accumulation. Note also that the right hemisphere (8) is compressed and shifting across the midline. This condition leads also to a compression of the right lateral ventricular system when compared to the left lateral ventricular system. (**B**) CT scan of a patient following a cerebral vascular accident involving major branches of the middle cerebral artery. The infarct has resulted in swelling of brain tissue altering its imaging characteristics. The infarcted tissue is encircled. Note that the infarcted tissue has swollen, producing the effects of a space-occupying lesion that has displaced the left hemisphere across the midline and distorted the lateral ventricular system. (**C**) CT scan with the vasculature enhanced showing an aneurysm associated with a branch of the middle cerebral artery. (**D**) CT scan of a patient showing the presence of a tumor (circled, *14*) located in the posterior cranial fossa. The tumor is impinging on the cerebellum, brain stem, and cranial nerves.

Computed Tomography (CT) and Magnetic Resonance Imaging (MRI) of the Brain and Spinal Cord

1. Temporal pole
2. Basilar artery
3. Hippocampus
4. Inferior horn of lateral ventricle
5. Ambient cistern
6. Pons
7. Fourth ventricle
8. Vermis of cerebellum
9. Cerebellum
10. Anterior horn of lateral ventricle
11. Insular cistern
12. Third ventricle
13. Trigone of lateral ventricle
14. Quadrigeminal cistern
15. Frontal pole
16. Septum pellucidum
17. Fornix
18. Interventricular foramen of Monro
19. Thalamus
20. Pineal
21. Posterior horn of lateral ventricle
22. Occipital pole
23. Interhemispheric fissure (falx)
24. Body of lateral ventricle

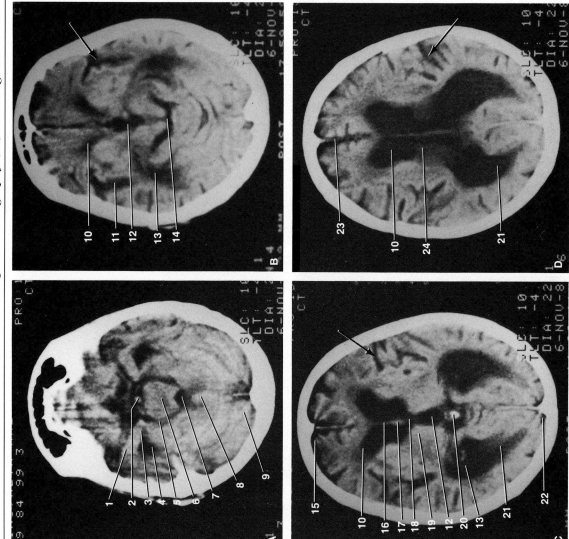

FIGURE 8-11.

(A–F) Series of CT scans (inferior to superior) showing cortical atrophy and hydrocephalus. Note that the fissures and sulci between gyri and lobes of the cerebral hemispheres are wide and filled with cerebrospinal fluid (*arrows*), suggesting that the cerebral cortex has atrophied. The lateral ventricular system has expanded to occupy the space.

Computed Tomography (CT) and Magnetic Resonance Imaging (MRI) of the Brain and Spinal Cord

23. Interhemispheric fissure (falx)
24. Body of lateral ventricle

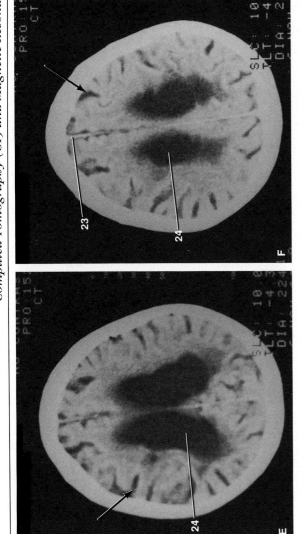

FIGURE 8-11   *Continued*

Atlas of the Human Brain, by Lothar Jennes,
Harold H. Traurig, and P. Michael Conn.
J. B. Lippincott Company, Philadelphia, © 1995.

Neuropathology of Common Diseases (Macroscopic and Microscopic)

chapter 9

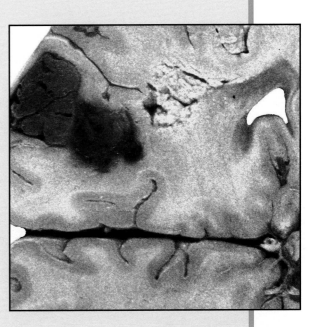

Neuropathology of Common Diseases (Macroscopic and Microscopic)

* the approximate position of the lateral sulcus;

+ the location of the central sulcus

1. Frontal pole
2. Temporal pole
3. Occipital pole
4. Cerebellum

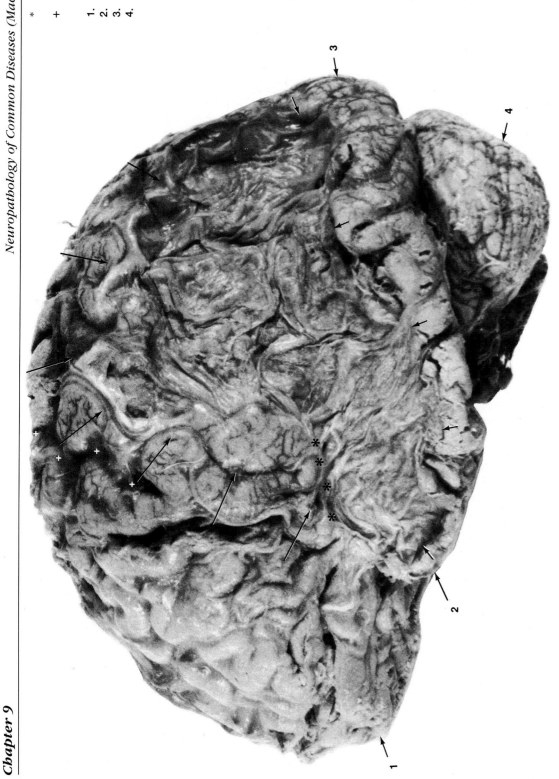

FIGURE 9-1.
Lateral view of left hemisphere from a person who suffered a loss of blood supply through the posterior distribution of the middle cerebral artery supplying the cortex of the parietal and lateral aspects of the occipital lobes. The boundaries of the cortical areas that lost their blood supply are indicated by the arrows. The person survived for at least several months following the loss of blood supply. During this period the degenerating cortical tissue was removed by glial cell action. The intact meninges lie on the surface of the degenerated cortex.

1. Fourth ventricle
2. Basilar artery

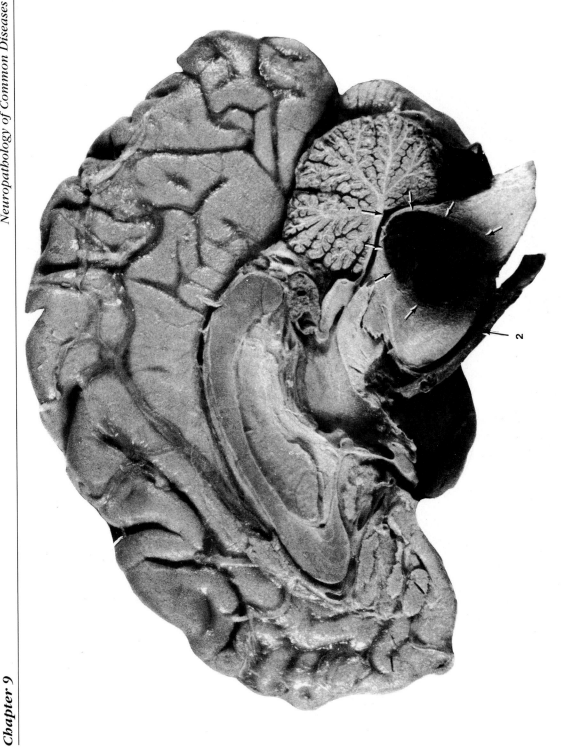

FIGURE 9-2.

Midsagittal view of right hemisphere showing a hemorrhagic infarct of the pons. Note that the extra-vasated blood has become a space-occupying lesion and is impinging on the fourth ventricle (*arrows*). This infarct is likely due to rupture of one or more feeder branches of the basilar artery, which supply the median vascular zone of the pons. This life-threatening cerebrovascular accident interrupts the blood supply to neurons and pathways that regulate such vital functions as respiratory rhythm and cardiovascular regulation.

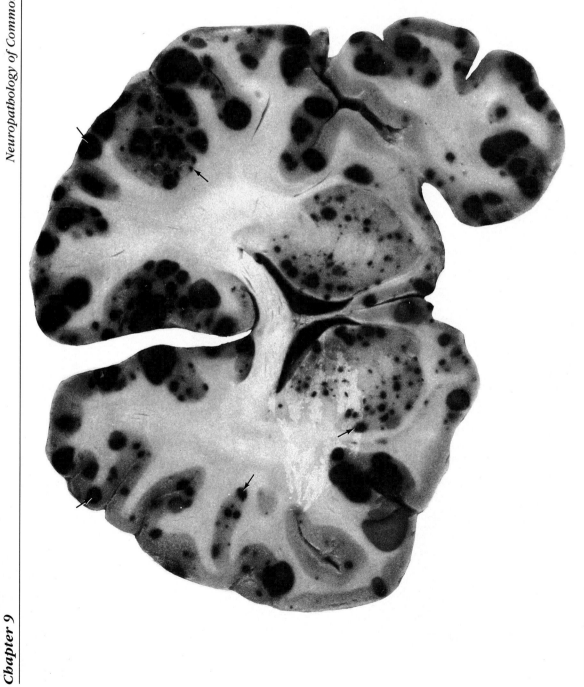

FIGURE 9-3.

A coronal section of the brain of a patient who had a malignant melanoma that metastasized to the brain as well as to other organs. In this case, the numerous tumors consist largely of cells containing melanin pigment and are easily recognized by their dark, round appearance (*arrows*). The spreading cancer cells tend to accumulate in areas of the central nervous system that have the greatest vascularity, in this case the cortical gray matter and basal ganglia.

Chapter 9

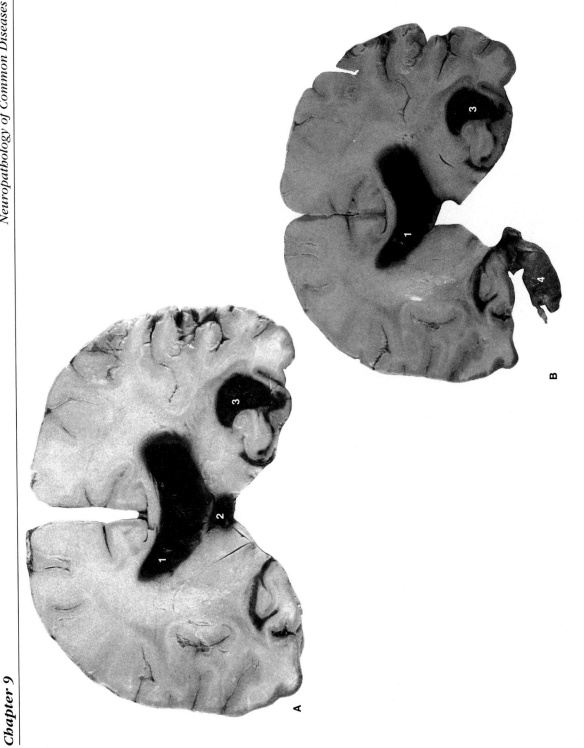

FIGURE 9-4.
(**A**) Coronal section of a brain that has had a vascular accident resulting in bleeding into the cerebroventricular system. The accumulated blood is seen dilating the bodies of the lateral ventricles (*1*), third ventricle (*2*), and one inferior horn of the lateral ventricle (*3*). (**B**) Another section of the same brain showing an aneurysm (*4*) associated with the cerebral vasculature.

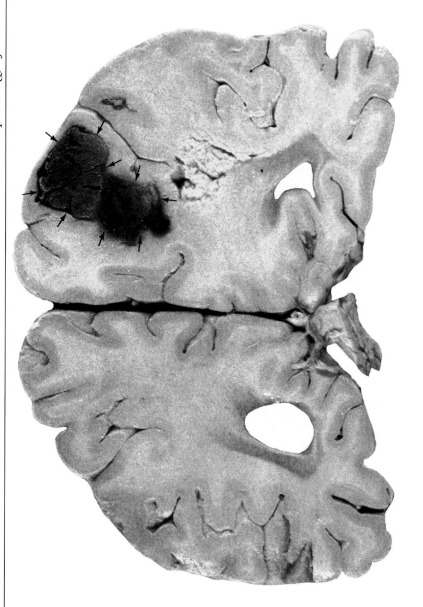

FIGURE 9-5.
Coronal section of the brain showing a malignant tumor that has metastasized from the kidney to the occipital lobe (*arrows*).

Chapter 9

1. Body of lateral ventricle
2. Inferior horn of lateral ventricle
3. Midbrain
4. Third ventricle
5. Pons

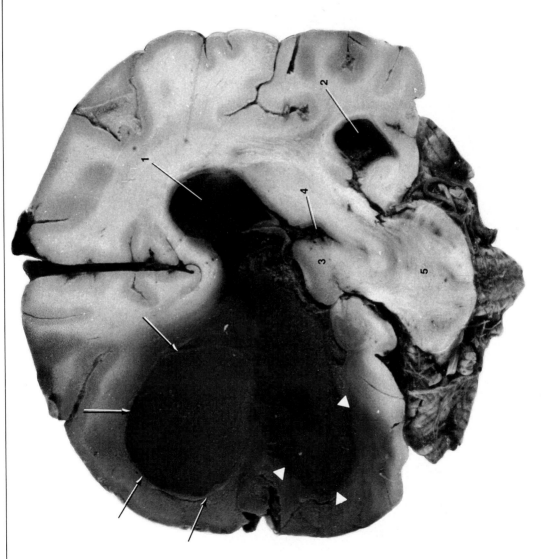

FIGURE 9-6.
Coronal section through the brain of a patient who died of a massive hemorrhagic cerebrovascular accident. There was an earlier episode of bleeding into the cerebral white matter, which appears to have organized a capsule surrounding the clotted blood (*arrows*). Subsequently, a second hemorrhagic episode occurred that resulted in additional accumulation of blood in the white matter (*arrowheads*) and the ventricular system. The accumulated blood formed a space-occupying lesion that resulted in a marked shift of the brainstem off the midline. Note the accumulated blood in the body (*1*) and inferior horn (*2*) of the lateral ventricle.

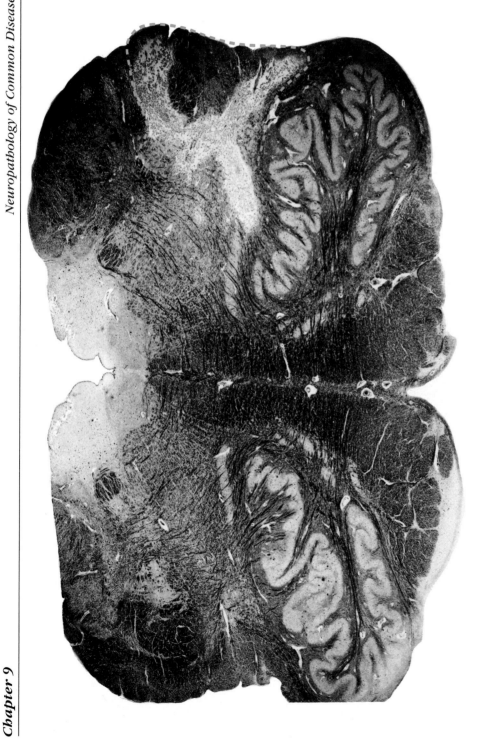

FIGURE 9-7.

Cross section of the medulla stained with a nerve fiber stain showing degeneration of the lateral vascular zone following a cerebrovascular accident of a nutrient branch of the posterior inferior cerebellar artery (PICA). The group of functional defects that often result from a cerebrovascular accident involving the PICA is referred to as the PICA, lateral medullary, or Wallenberg syndrome.

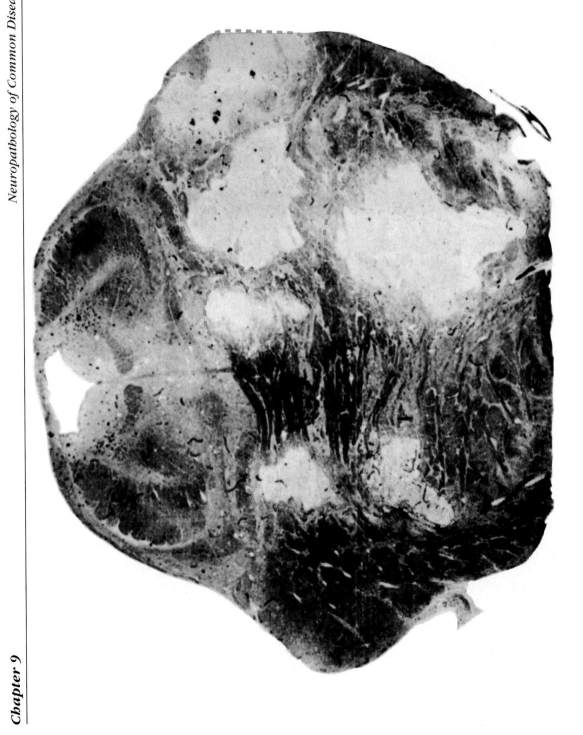

FIGURE 9-8.
Cross section through the rostral pons of a patient with multiple sclerosis (nerve fiber stain). Scar tissue occupies the area of the brain stem affected. These accumulations of scar tissue are referred to as plaques.

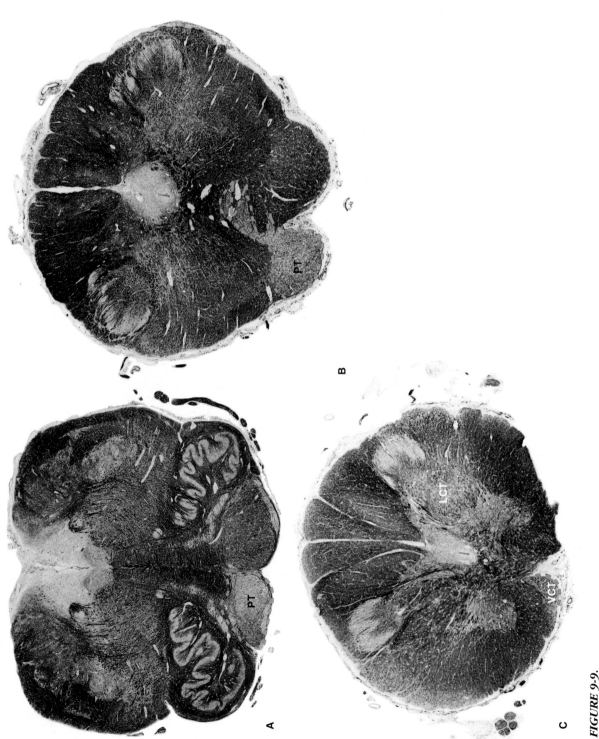

FIGURE 9-9.

Series of cross sections of (**A,B**) brain stem and the upper cervical spinal cord (**C**) of a patient who had a cerebrovascular accident of the internal capsule. The voluntary motor pathway (pyramidal tract, PT) axons have been interrupted. Their degeneration is evident in the ipsilateral pyramid (pyramid (**A**) and motor decussation (**B**) in the brain stem and in the contralateral corticospinal tract (LCT) and ipsilateral ventral corticospinal tract (VCT) in the upper cervical spinal cord (**C**).

Chapter 9

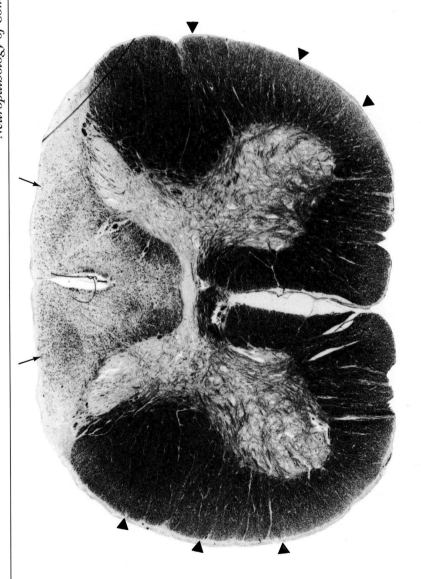

FIGURE 9-10.
Cross section of the lumosacral spinal cord stained with a nerve fiber stain from a patient who had syphilis that affected the nervous system. Degeneration of the fiber tracts of the dorsal columns is evident (*arrows*). There is also some degeneration in the region occupied by the spinocerebellar tracts (*arrowheads*).

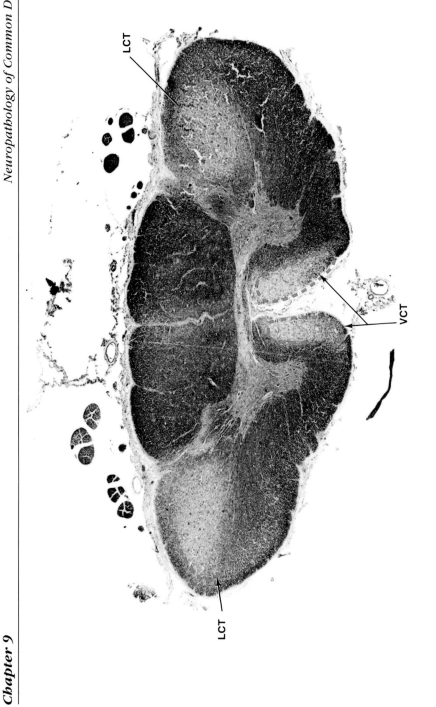

FIGURE 9-11.

Cross section of the spinal cord stained with a nerve fiber stain from a patient who suffered an interruption of both pyramidal tracts in the pons. Degeneration is evident in the lateral (LCT) and ventral (VCT) corticospinal tracts.

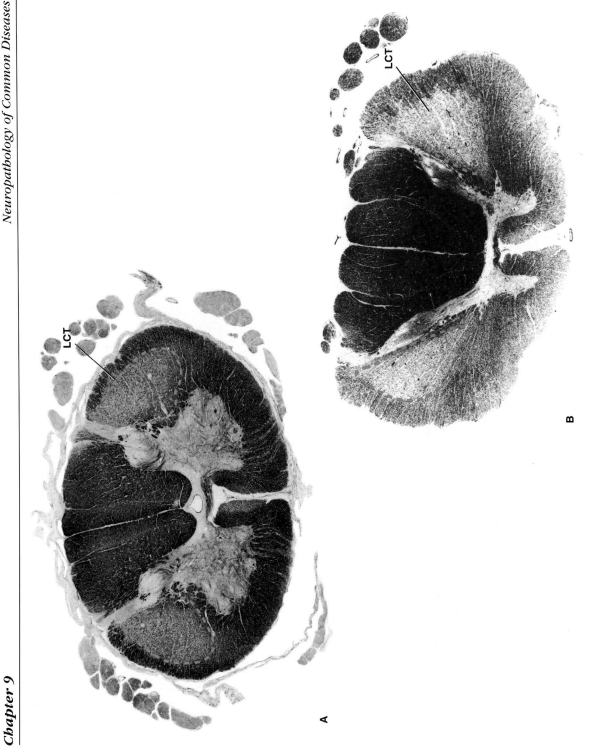

FIGURE 9-12.

Cross sections of the cervical (**A**) and upper thoracic (**B**) spinal cord from a patient with amyotrophic lateral sclerosis (ALS). Degeneration of several neural pathways—for example, the lateral corticospinal tract (LCT)—is evident, especially in the thoracic region.

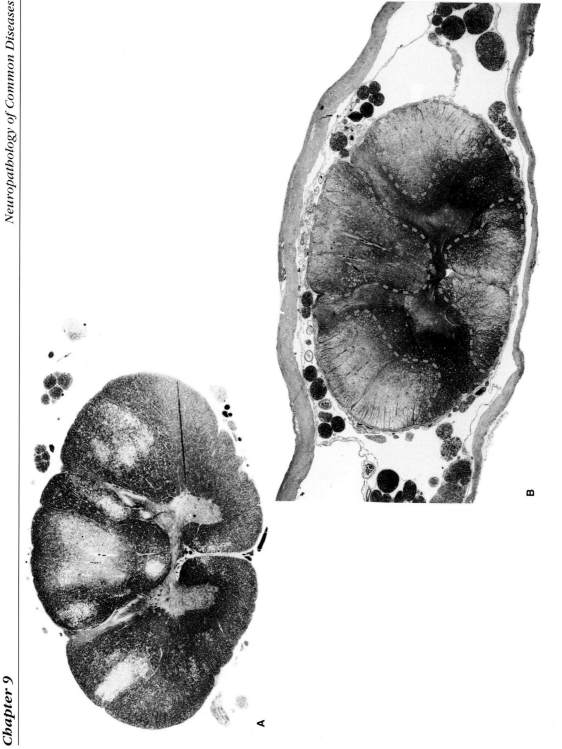

FIGURE 9-13.

Cross section of the thoracic spinal cords of two patients with posterior lateral sclerosis or subacute combined degeneration of the spinal cord. The spinal cord in **B** is more affected. This degeneration is thought to be the result of disturbances in vitamin B_{12} absorption. The unstained regions of the spinal cord white matter reflect degenerated nerve fibers *(outlined by a dashed line)*.

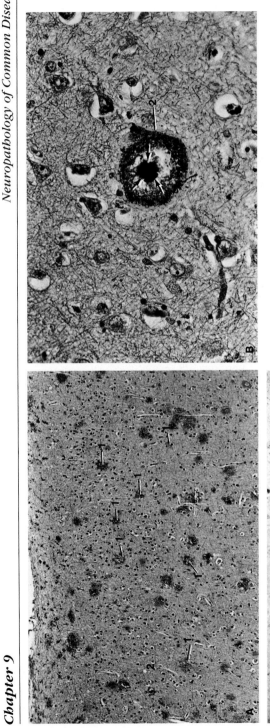

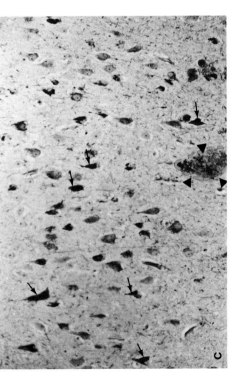

FIGURE 9-14.

Frontal cortex area 9 of a patient who was diagnosed with Alzheimer's disease showing both dementia and neuropathological signs (Bielschowsky silver stain). Numerous diffuse plaques (*1*) and neuritic plaques with ameloid core (*2*) are concentrated in laminas 3 and 5 (**A**). (**B**) High magnification of a neuritic plaque with ameloid core (*arrows*). (**C**) High magnification of neurofibrillary tangles (*arrows*) and diffuse plaques (*arrowheads*).

Atlas of the Human Brain, by Lothar Jennes,
Harold H. Traurig, and P. Michael Conn.
J. B. Lippincott Company, Philadelphia, © 1995.

H*istology of the Central*
Nervous System

c h a p t e r 10

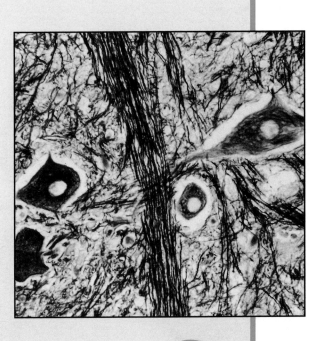

1. Cell soma of a pyramidal cell
2. Apical dendrite
3. Basal dendrite
4. Initial portion of axon
5. Cell soma of neuron in the striatum
6. Dendrite with spines

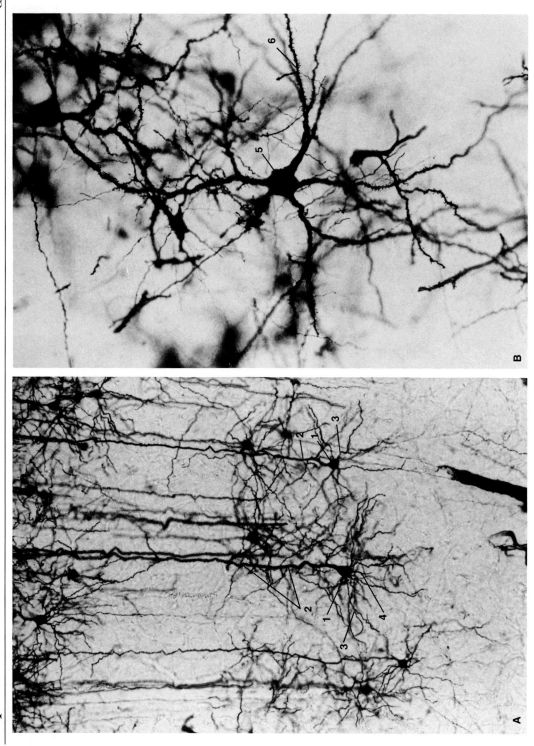

FIGURE 10-1.
Light micrographs of (**A**) the cerebral cortex and (**B**) striatum showing neurons after Golgi-Kopsch silver impregnation.

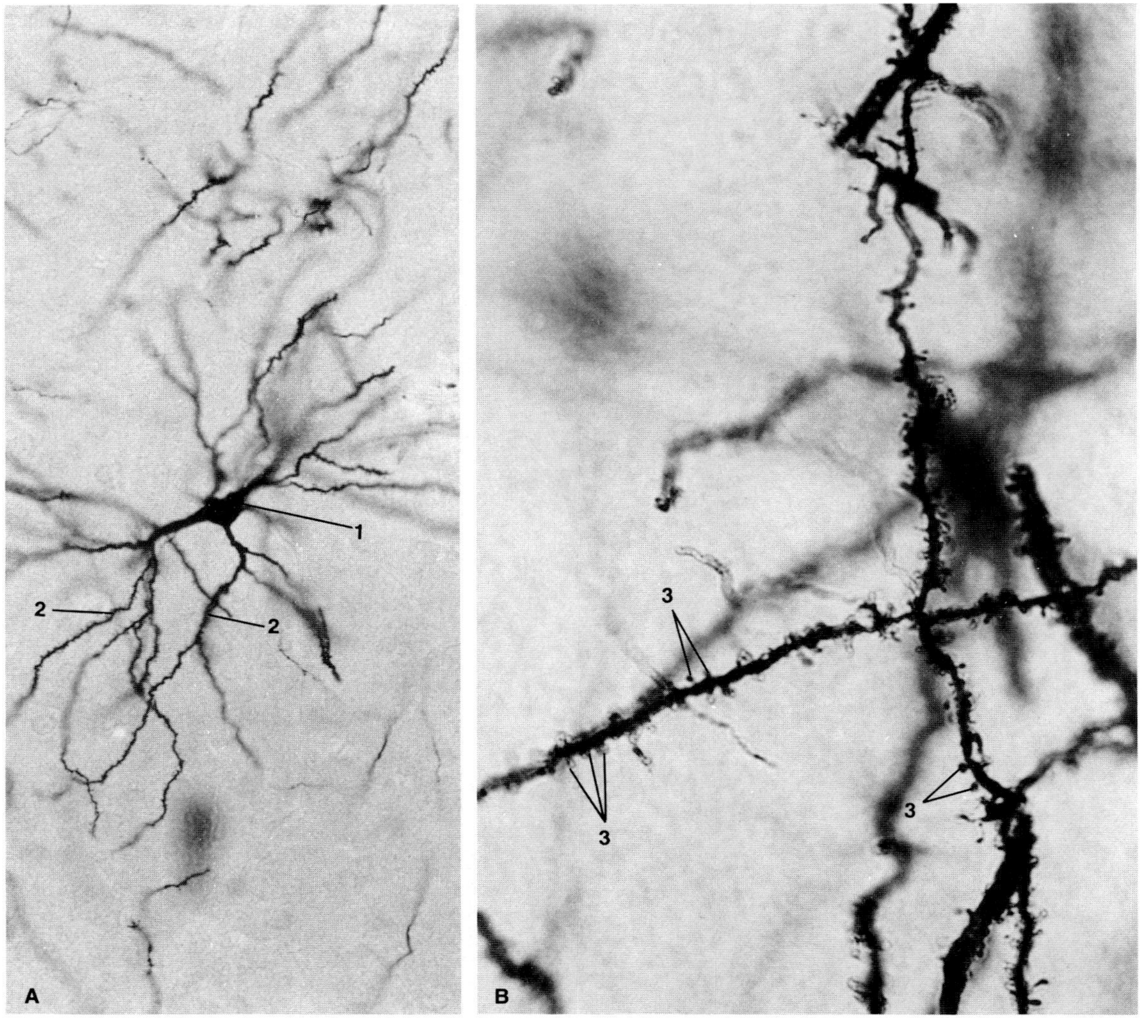

1. Cell soma
2. Dendrites
3. Dendritic spines

FIGURE 10-2.

Light micrographs of a neuron in the striatum (**A**) and high magnification of dendrites in the cerebral cortex (**B**) after Golgi-Kopsch silver impregnation.

Histology of the Central Nervous System

1. Motor neuron
2. Nissl substance
3. Nucleus
4. Nucleolus
5. Axon hillock
6. Proximal dendrite
7. Glia cell nuclei
8. Cross section through myelinated axons

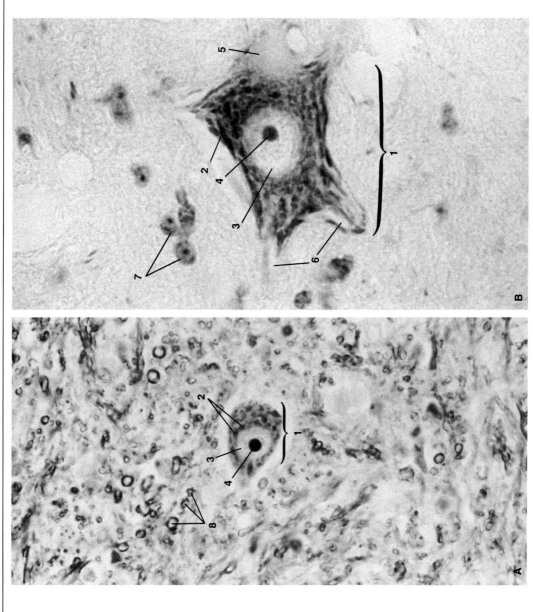

FIGURE 10-3.

Motor neurons in the spinal cord stained with Nissl and Luxol fast blue (**A**) and with Nissl alone (**B**). The dark staining circular profiles in **A** represent the myelin surrounding unstained axons.

1. Motor neuron
2. Nucleus
3. Neurofilament bundles
4. Purkinje neuron
5. Nucleolus
6. Perikaryon
7. Axon terminals of basket cells
8. Molecular layer
9. Granule layer

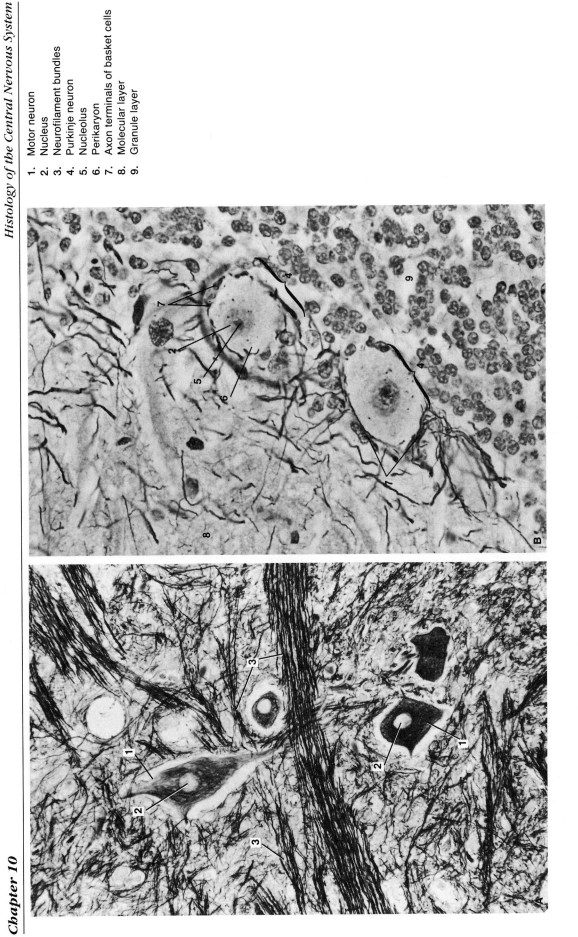

FIGURE 10-4.

Light micrographs of (**A**) a motor neuron in the spinal cord stained with a Bielschowsky silver stain and (**B**) a Purkinje neuron in the cerebellum stained with Bodian stain.

1. Purkinje neurons
2. Molecular layer
3. Granule layer
4. Golgi cells
5. Dendrites of Purkinje neurons
6. Axons of basket cells

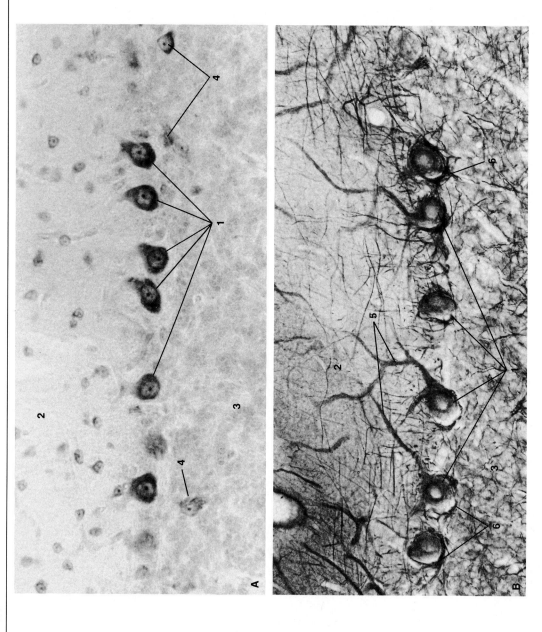

FIGURE 10-5.
Purkinje neurons in the cerebellum stained with toluidine blue (**A**) and with Huber-Guild silver impregnation (**B**).

1. Glial cell soma
2. Glial cell processes

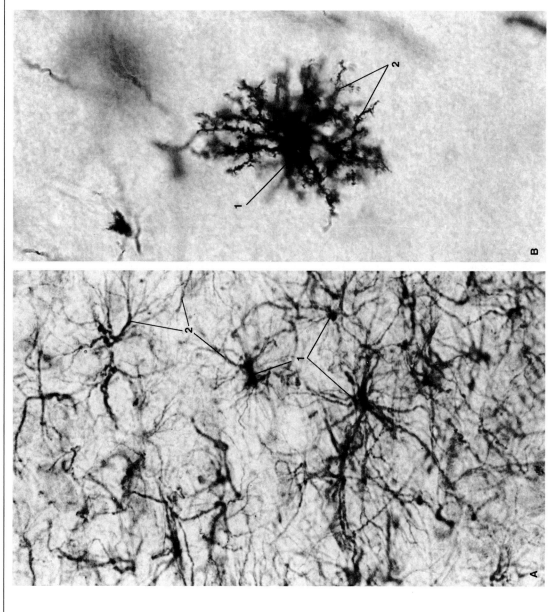

FIGURE 10-6.
Protoplasmic astrocytes stained immunohistochemically with antibodies to glial fibrillary acetic protein (**A**) and with a Golgi silver impregnation (**B**).

1. Cell soma
2. Cell processes
3. White matter (corpus callosum)

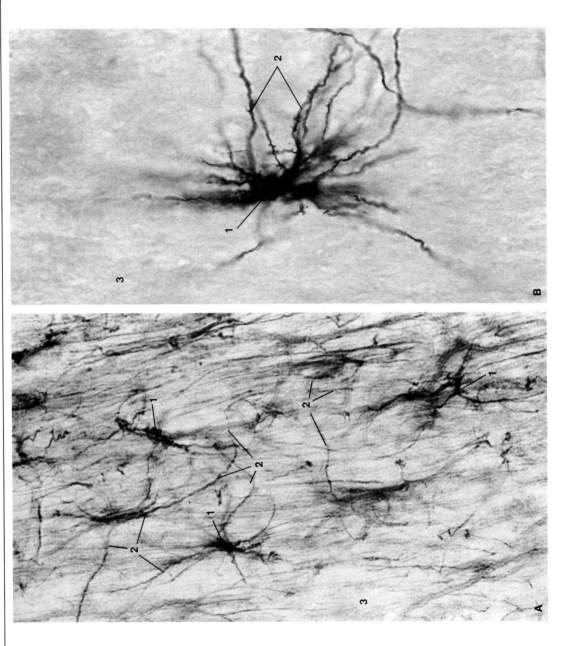

FIGURE 10-7.
Fibrous astrocytes stained immunohistochemically with antibodies to glial fibrillary acetic protein (**A**) and with Golgi silver impregnation (**B**).

1. Cell soma of a fibrous astrocyte
2. Cell processes ("end feet" surrounding blood vessel)
3. Blood vessel
4. Cell soma of a microglia cell
5. Cell processes of a microglia cell

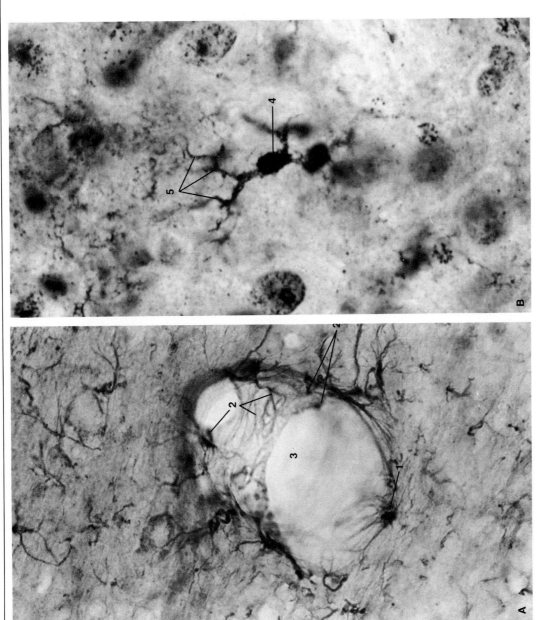

FIGURE 10-8.
Light micrograph of (**A**) a fibrous astrocyte stained with Cajal silver stain and (**B**) a microglia cell stained with Del Rio Hortega silver stain.

Atlas of the Human Brain, by Lothar Jennes, Harold H. Traurig, and P. Michael Conn. J. B. Lippincott Company, Philadelphia. © 1995.

Histology of the Peripheral Nervous System

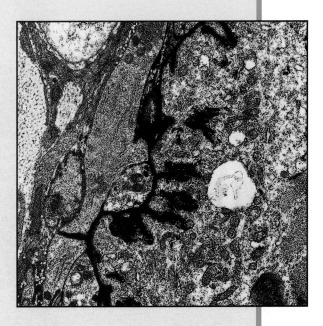

chapter 11

1. Nucleolus of ganglion cell
2. Nucleus of ganglion cell
3. Cytoplasm of ganglion cell
4. Nerve fiber bundle
5. Inner circular smooth muscle layer of the digestive tract
6. Outer longitudinal smooth muscle layer of the digestive tract

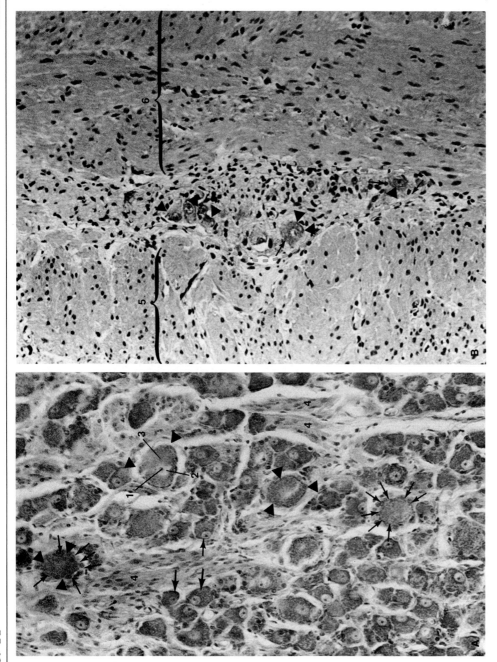

FIGURE 11-1.

Histological sections through (**A**) a sensory ganglion (dorsal root ganglion) and (**B**) an autonomic motor ganglion (Auerbach's plexus).

In the dorsal root ganglion, the diameters of the neuron vary substantially. In general, the larger neurons (*arrowheads*) give rise to large-diameter fibers associated with tactile and proprioceptive sensation, whereas the smaller neurons (*large arrows*) give rise to small-diameter fibers which are non- or only slightly myelinated. These fibers convey nociceptive sensation. All neurons in the dorsal root ganglion are covered by satellite cells (*small arrows*). Luxol fast blue–nuclear red stain.

In Auerbach's plexus the ganglion cells are smaller in diameter and multipolar (*arrowheads*) and the satellite cells (*arrows*) are less numerous when compared to the sensory ganglia. Hematoxylin-eosin stain.

1. Epineurium
2. Perineurium
3. Myelinated axons
4. Vasa vasorum

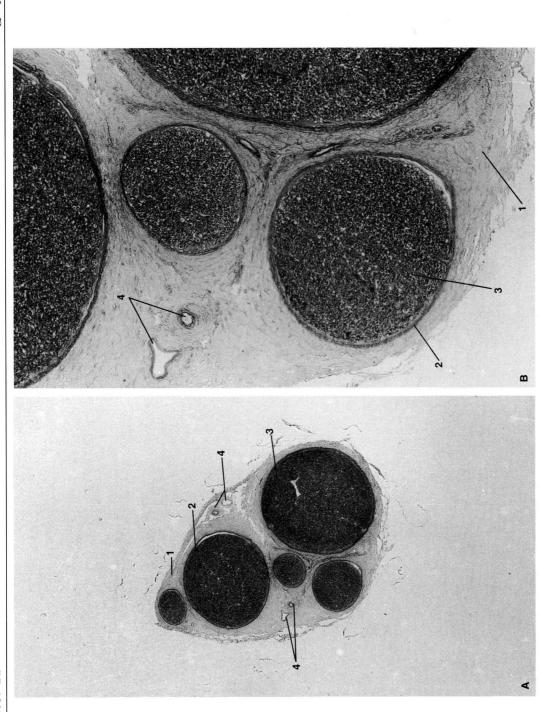

FIGURE 11-2.
Cross sections of a peripheral nerve at low (**A**) and high (**B**) magnification; fast green staining.

1. Adipose cells in the epineurium
2. Perineurium
3. Endoneurium
4. Individual myelinated axons
5. Node of Ranvier
6. Cleft of Schmitt-Lantermann

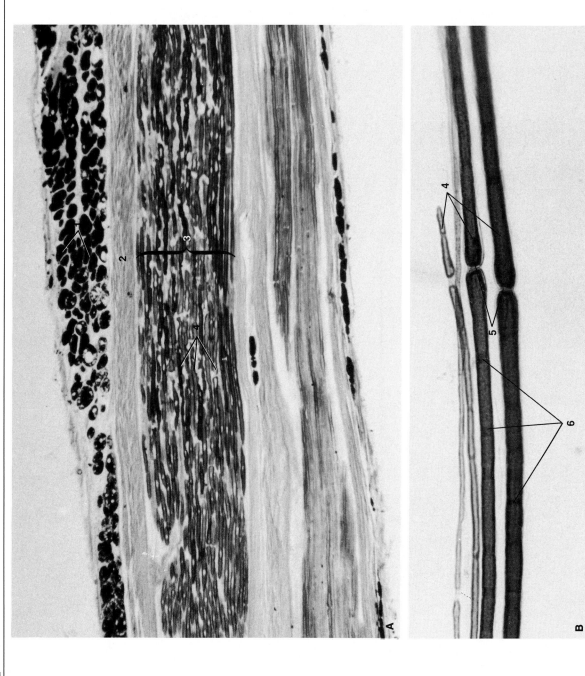

FIGURE 11-3.

Longitudinal section (**A**) and tease preparation (**B**) of a peripheral nerve; osmium tetroxide stain.

154

1. Neurovascular bundle
2. Peripheral nerve
3. Perineural lymphatic vessel
4. Arteriole
5. Venule
6. Myelin sheath
7. Nucleus of Schwann cell
8. Axon (surrounded by myelin sheath)
9. Endoneurium
10. Perineurium

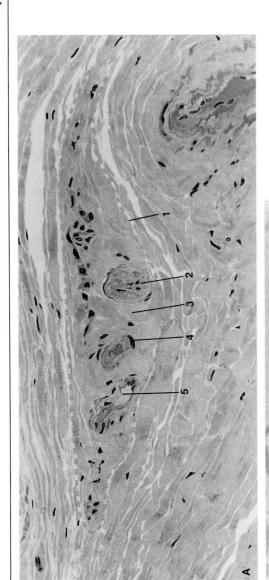

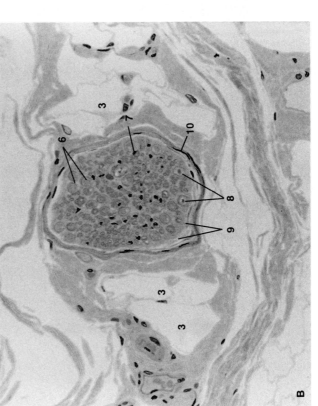

FIGURE 11-4.

Neuro-vascular bundle (**A**) and small peripheral nerve with perineural lymphatic vessels (**B**); hematoxylin–eosin stain.

1. Intramuscular nerve
2. Motor end plates
3. Myelinated axons
4. Skeletal muscle fibers
5. Axon terminal
6. Schwann cell
7. Myelinated axon
8. Primary synaptic cleft (stained for acetylcholinesterase)
9. Secondary synaptic cleft (stained for acetylcholinesterase)
10. Junctional folds in sarcolemma
11. Nucleus of skeletal muscle fiber
12. Myofibrils

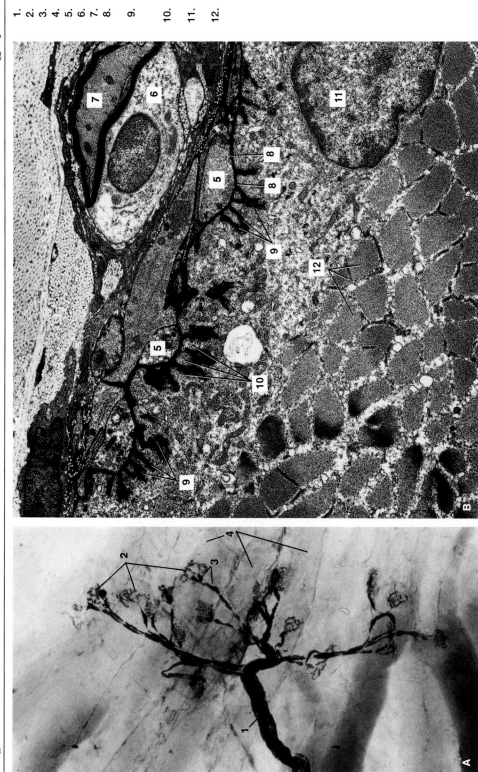

FIGURE 11-5.

Motor end plates as seen with the light microscope on a whole-mount preparation after silver impregnation (**A**) and with the electron microscope after staining for acetylcholinesterase (**B**).

Histology of the Peripheral Nervous System

1. Connective tissue capsule
2. Capsular space
3. Intrafusal nuclear chain fibers
4. Intrafusal nuclear bag fibers
5. Extrafusal muscle fibers

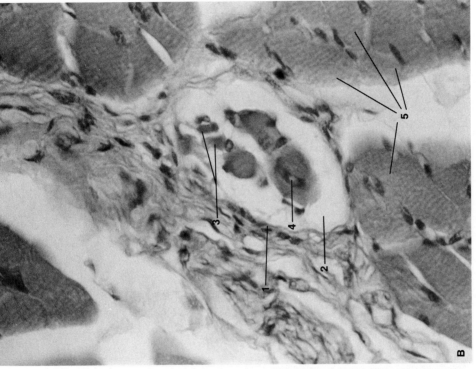

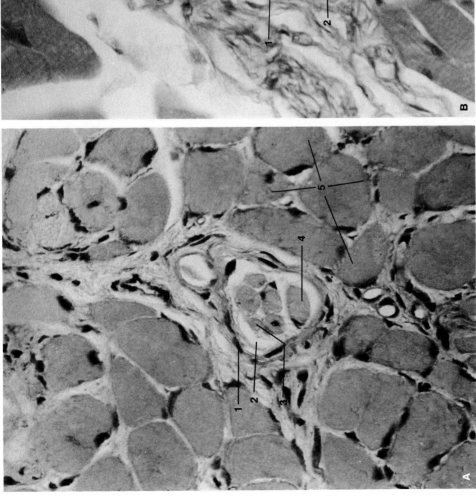

FIGURE 11-6.
Light micrographs of muscular tissue showing two cross sections of muscle spindles; hematoxylin–eosin stain.

1. Scala vestibuli
2. Scala media (cochlear duct)
3. Scala tympani
4. Spiral ligament
5. Cochlear nerve
6. Vestibular membrane (Reissner's membrane)
7. Organ of Corti
8. Outer bony wall of cochlea
9. Spiral ganglion
10. Modilus
11. Stria vascularis
12. Vestibular lip
13. Tectorial membrane
14. Inner sulcus cells
15. Inner sulcus
16. Inner hair cells
17. Inner phalangeal cells
18. Inner pillar cells
19. Inner tunnel
20. Outer pillar cells
21. Outer tunnel
22. Outer phalangeal cells
23. Outer hair cells
24. Basilar membrane
25. Bundles of dendrites of the spiral ganglion primary afferent neurons

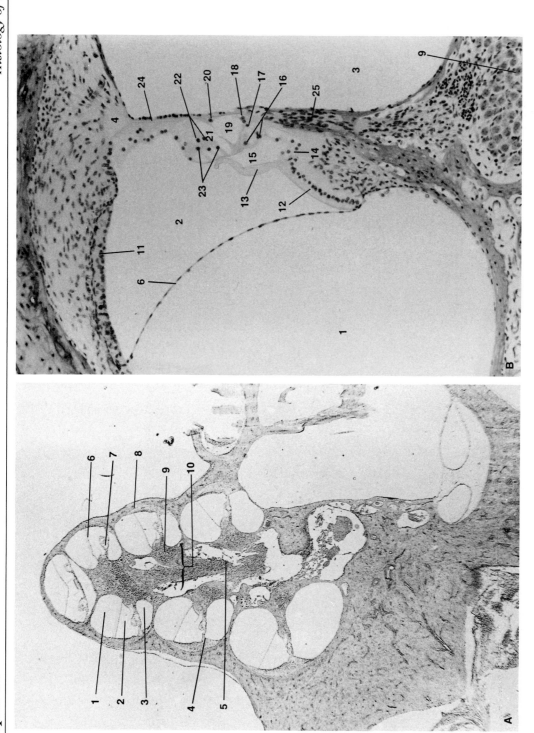

FIGURE 11-7.
Low power micrograph of the cochlear (**A**) and high magnification micrograph of the organ of Corti (**B**); hematoxylin–eosin stain.

1. Perilymphatic space lined by simple squameous epithelium (*arrows*)
2. Ampulla of a semicircular duct
3. Crista
4. Macula utriculi

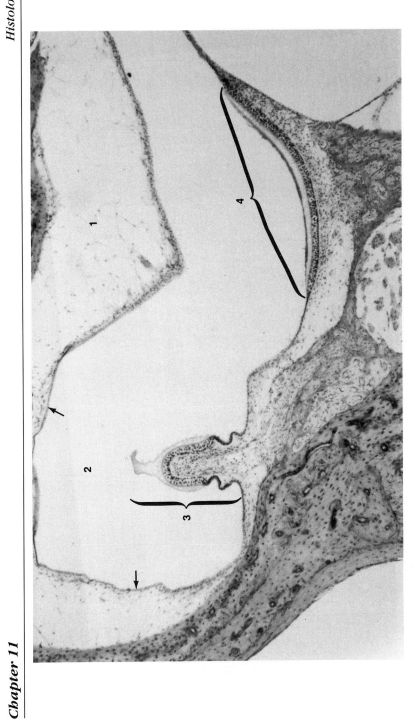

FIGURE 11-8.
Low power micrograph showing the sensory organs of the vestibular system; hematoxylin–eosin stain.

1. Ampulla of a semicircular duct
   filled with endolymph
2. Cupula
3. Hair cells
4. Supporting cells
5. Vestibular nerve fibers
   (myelinated)
6. Utricle
7. Otoliths
8. Otolitic membrane
9. Bone of the bony labyrinth

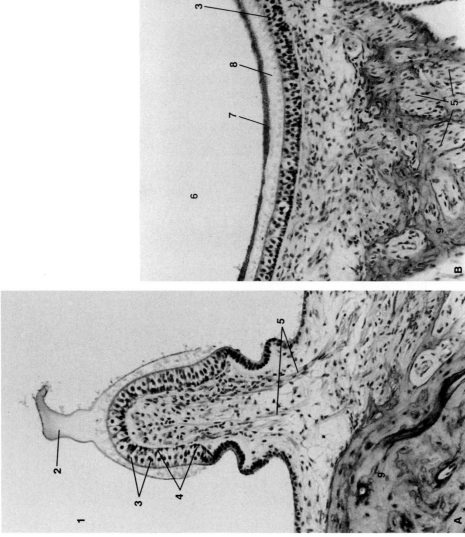

FIGURE 11-9.

Higher magnification of the sensory organs of the vestibular system showing a crista (**A**) and a macula
(**B**); hematoxylin–eosin stain.

Histology of the Peripheral Nervous System

1. Pigment epithelium
2. Layer of rods and cones
3. Outer limiting membrane
4. Outer nuclear layer
5. Outer plexiform layer
6. Inner nuclear layer
7. Inner plexiform layer
8. Ganglion cell layer
9. Nerve fiber layer
10. Inner limiting membrane
11. Vitreous chamber
12. Sclera
13. Choroid
14. Cones
15. Rods
16. Nuclei of cone cells
17. Nuclei of rod cells

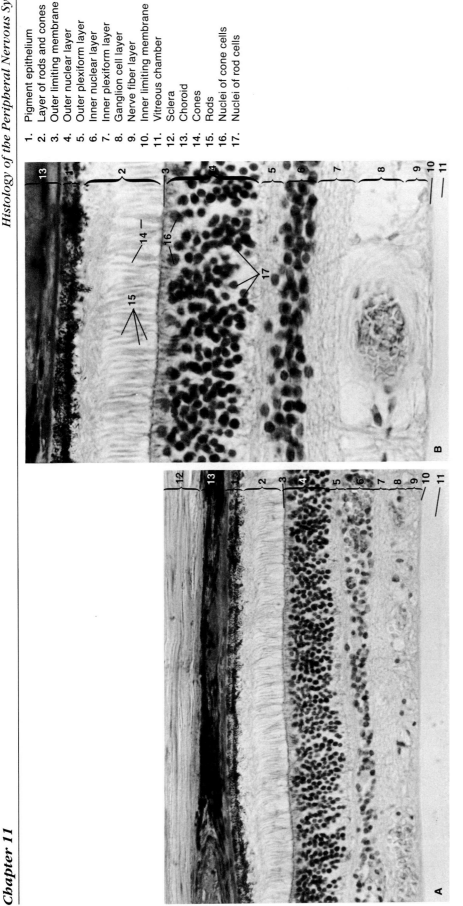

FIGURE 11-10.
Light micrographs of the retina at low (**A**) and high (**B**) magnification; hematoxylin–eosin stain.

1. Pigment epithelium
2. Layer of rods and cones
3. Outer limiting membrane
4. Outer nuclear layer
5. Outer plexiform layer
6. Inner nuclear layer
7. Inner plexiform layer
8. Ganglion cell layer
9. Nerve fiber layer
10. Inner limiting membrane
11. Fovea centralis (macula lutea)
12. Cone cells
13. Optic disc
14. Central blood vessel
15. Lamina cribrosa
16. Optic nerve
17. Pial sheath
18. Dural sheath
19. Choroid
20. Sclera
21. Perioptic subarachnoid space

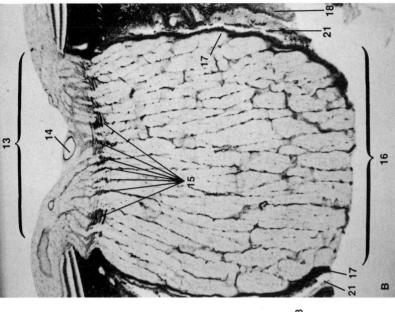

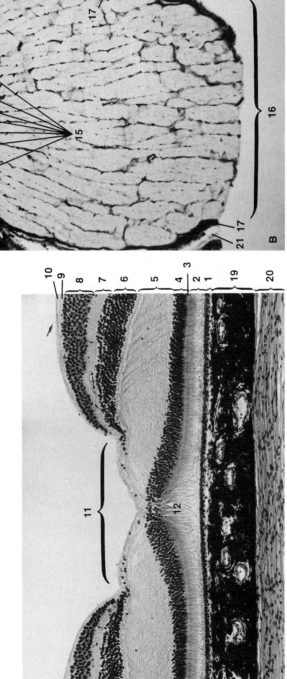

FIGURE 11-11.

Light micrographs of the fovea centralis (**A**) and the optic disc (**B**); hematoxylin–eosin stain.

1. Dermal papilla
2. Schwann cells
3. Capillary
4. Non-myelinated axons
5. Myelinated axons

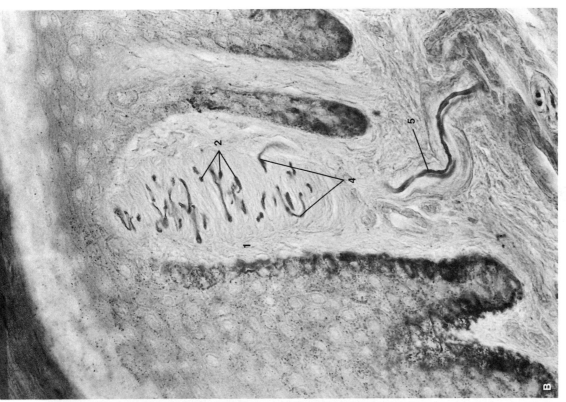

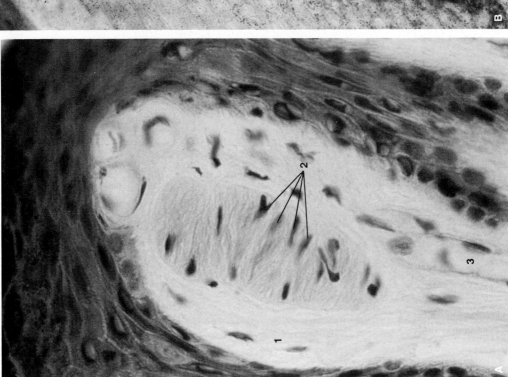

FIGURE 11-12.

Light micrographs of Meissner's corpuscles, which are tactile receptors in the papillary layer of the dermis. (**A**) shows hematoxylin–eosin stain; (**B**) shows silver impregnation.

1. Hypodermis
2. Connective tissue capsule
3. Connective tissue lamellae
4. Inner core
5. Schwann cells

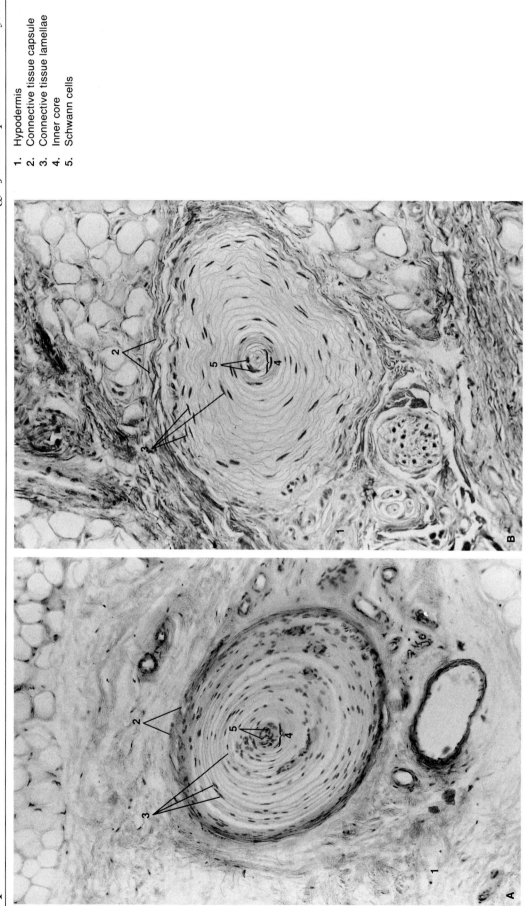

FIGURE 11-13.

Light micrographs of Pacinian corpuscles, which are very sensitive to vibration. (**A**) shows a hematoxylin–eosin stain; (**B**) shows silver impregnation.

Atlas of the Human Brain, by Lothar Jennes, Harold H. Traurig, and P. Michael Conn. J. B. Lippincott Company, Philadelphia, © 1995.

Ultrastructure of the Central and Peripheral Nervous Systems

c h a p t e r 12

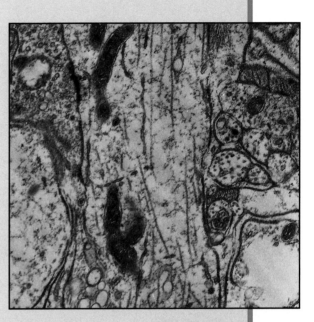

Ultrastructure of the Central and Peripheral Nervous Systems

1. Nucleus
2. Nucleolus
3. Nuclear envelope
4. Rough endoplasmic reticulum
   (Nissl body)
5. Golgi apparatus
6. Secondary lysosome
7. Mitochondrium
8. Plasma membrane
9. Astrocyte
10. Oligodendrocyte

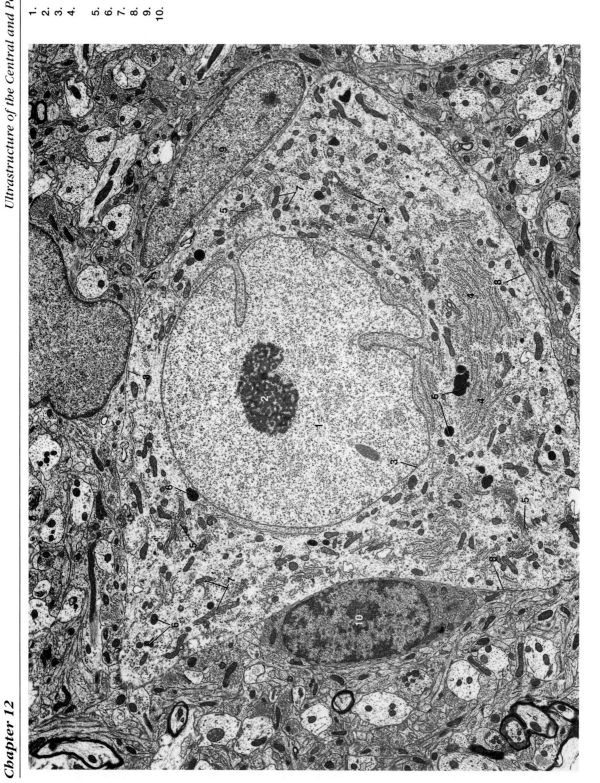

FIGURE 12-1.
Pyramidal neuron in the hippocampus.

Ultrastructure of the Central and Peripheral Nervous Systems

1. Nucleus
2. Nucleolus
3. Nuclear envelope
4. Mitochondrium
5. Golgi apparatus
6. Axo-somatic synapse

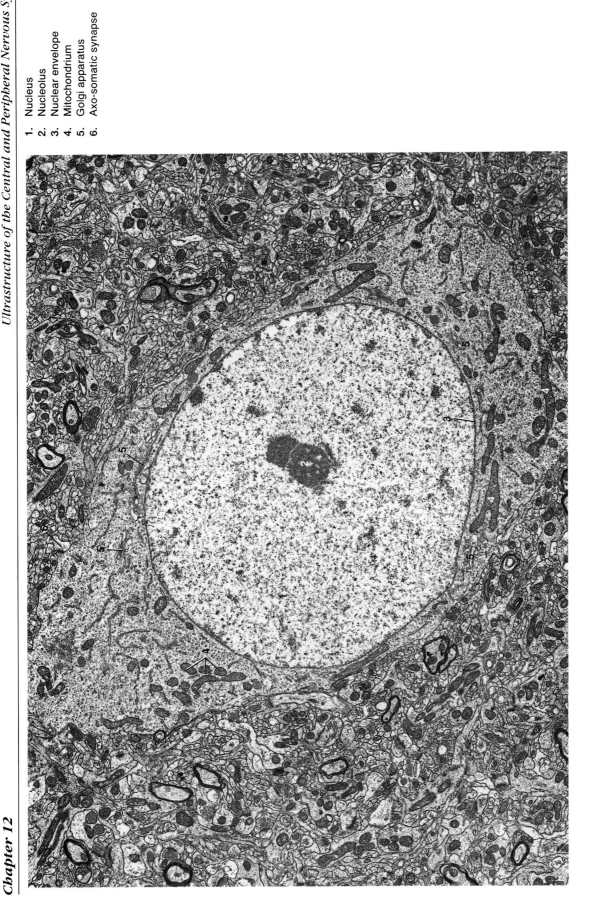

FIGURE 12-2.
Neuron in the cerebral cortex.

Ultrastructure of the Central and Peripheral Nervous Systems

1. Nucleus
2. Nucleolus
3. Nuclear envelope
4. Rough endoplasmic reticulum
   (Nissl body)
5. Golgi apparatus
6. Neurosecretory vesicle
7. Mitochondrium
8. Secondary lysosome
9. Plasma membrane
10. Capillary
11. Continuous endothelium

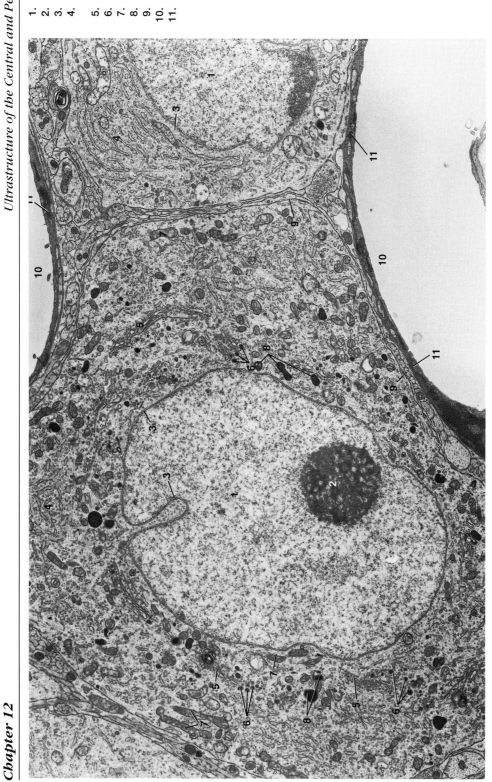

FIGURE 12-3.
Hypothalamic neurosecretory neuron.

Ultrastructure of the Central and Peripheral Nervous Systems

1. Dendrite
2. Neurotubule
3. Neurofilament
4. Mitochondrium
5. Axon
6. Axo-dendritic synapse
7. Myelin

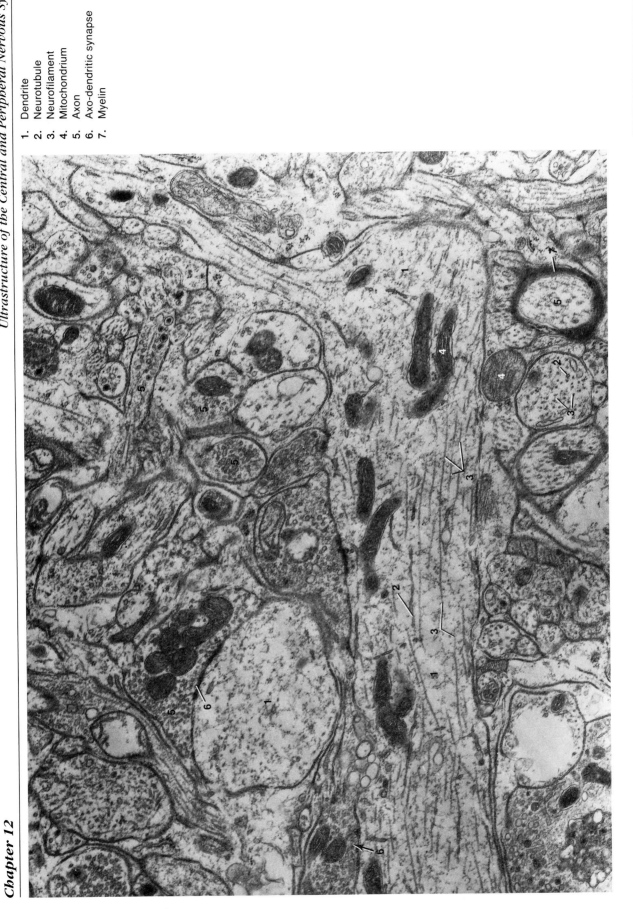

FIGURE 12-4.
Neuropil in the brain stem.

Ultrastructure of the Central and Peripheral Nervous Systems

1. Dendrite
2. Neurotubule
3. Neurofilament
4. Mitochondrium
5. Axon
6. Axo-dendritic synapse
7. Myelin
8. Dense core vesicle

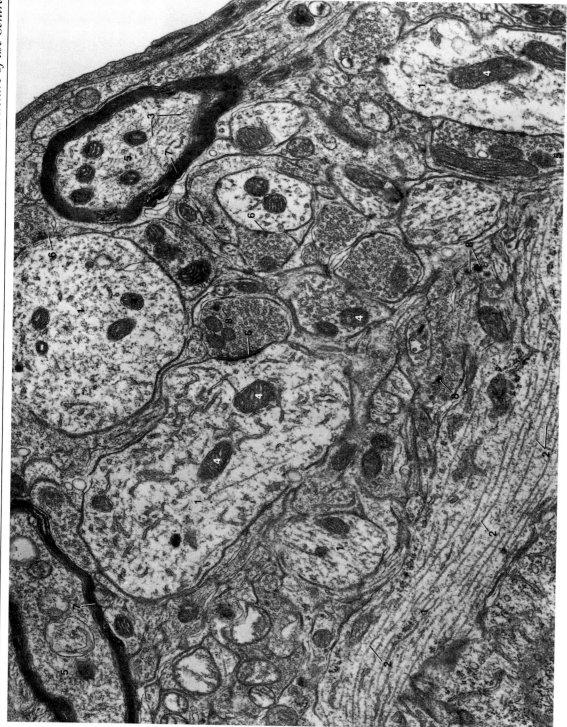

FIGURE 12-5.
Neuropil in the brain stem.

Ultrastructure of the Central and Peripheral Nervous Systems

1. Dendrite
2. Dendritic spine
3. Mitochondrium
4. Synaptic complex
5. Axon terminal with synaptic vesicles

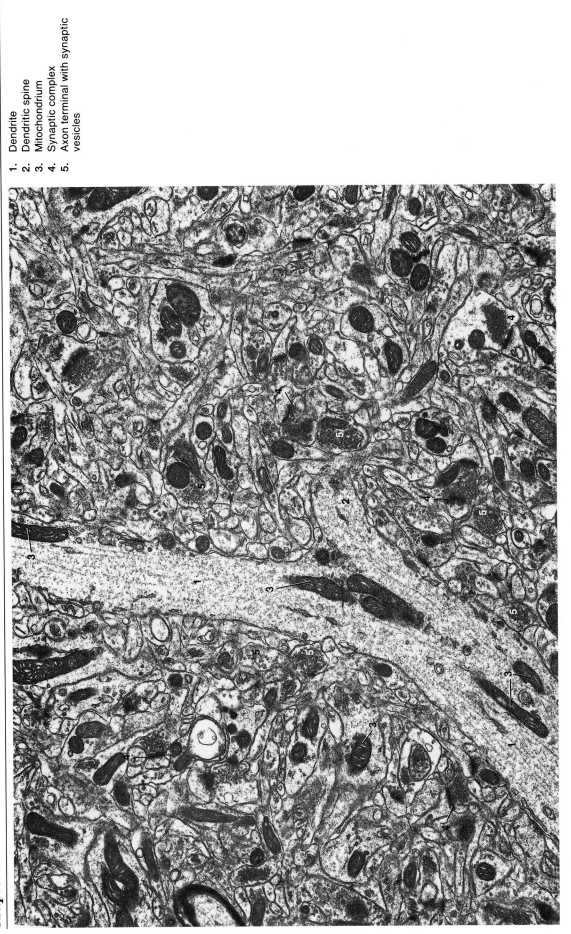

FIGURE 12-6.
Neuropil in the cerebral cortex.

Ultrastructure of the Central and Peripheral Nervous Systems

1. Axon
2. Dendrite
3. Synaptic vesicles
4. Axo-dendritic synapse
5. Presynaptic membrane
6. Synaptic cleft
7. Postsynaptic membrane
8. Neurotubules
9. Neurofilaments

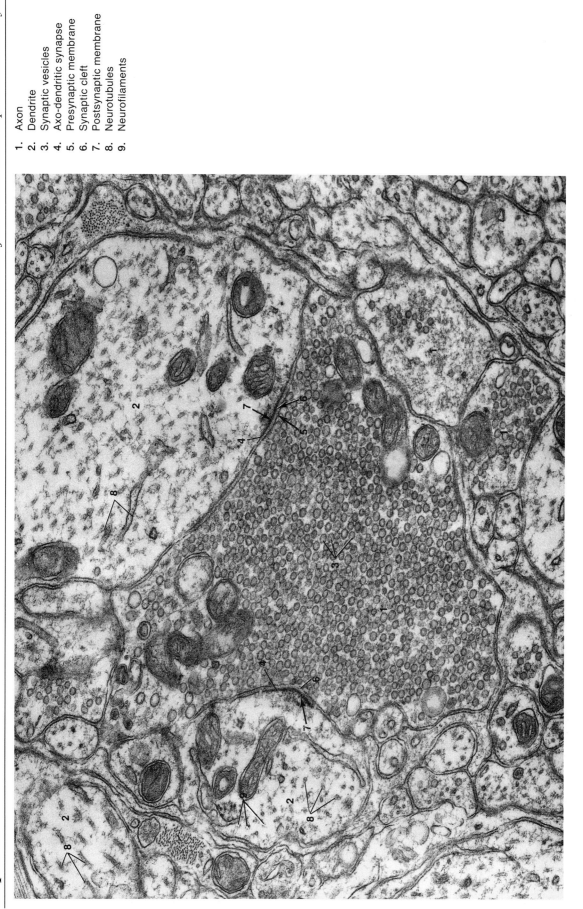

FIGURE 12-7.
Axo-dendritic synapse.

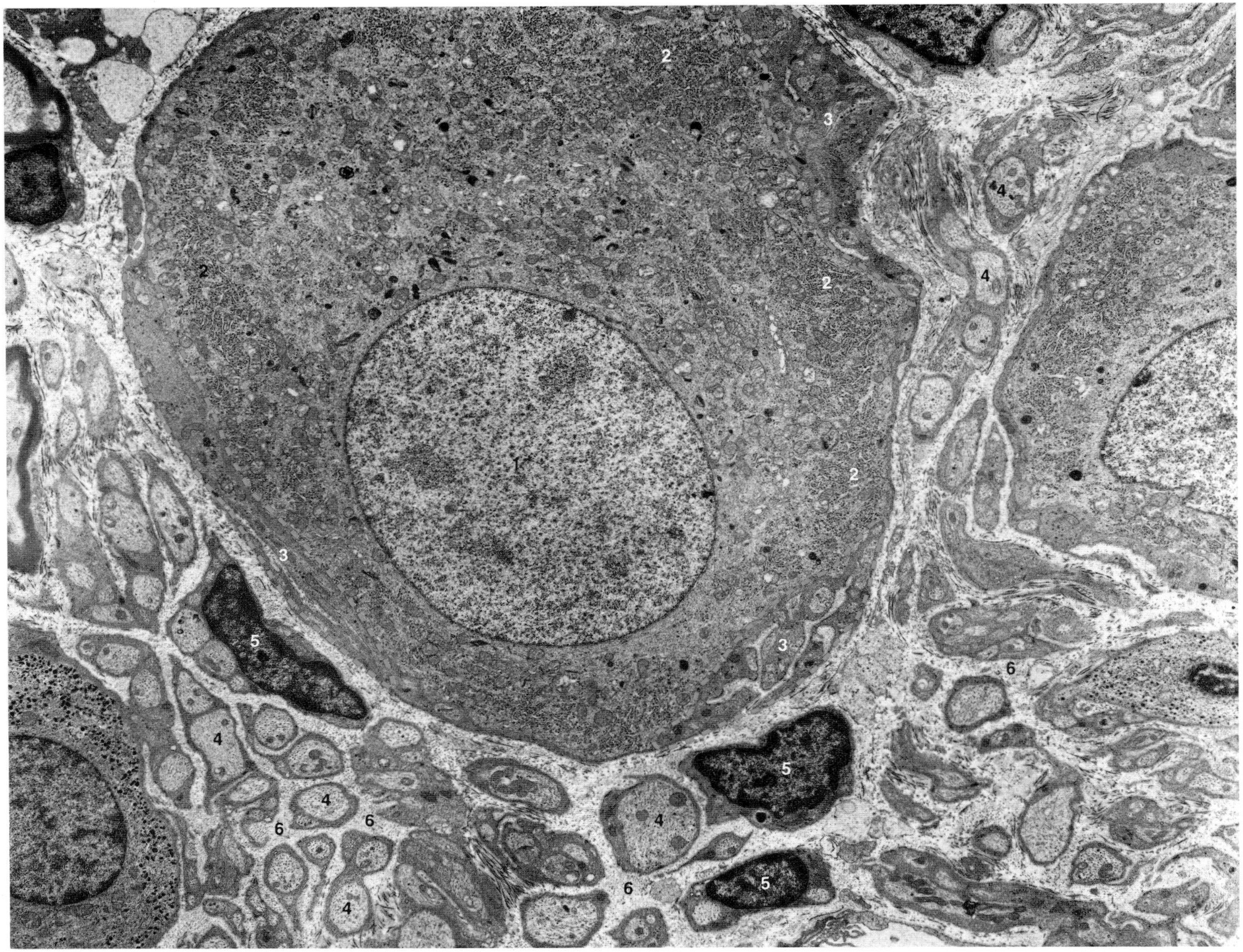

Ultrastructure of the Central and Peripheral Nervous Systems

1. Nucleus
2. Rough endoplasmic reticulum (Nissl body)
3. Satellite cell
4. Unmyelinated axon
5. Schwann cell
6. Endoneurium

FIGURE 12-8.
Ganglion cell of the autonomic nervous system (paracervical ganglion).

Ultrastructure of the Central and Peripheral Nervous Systems

1. Motor neuron
2. Nucleus
3. Schwann cell
4. Satellite cell
5. Unmyelinated axon
6. Endoneurium

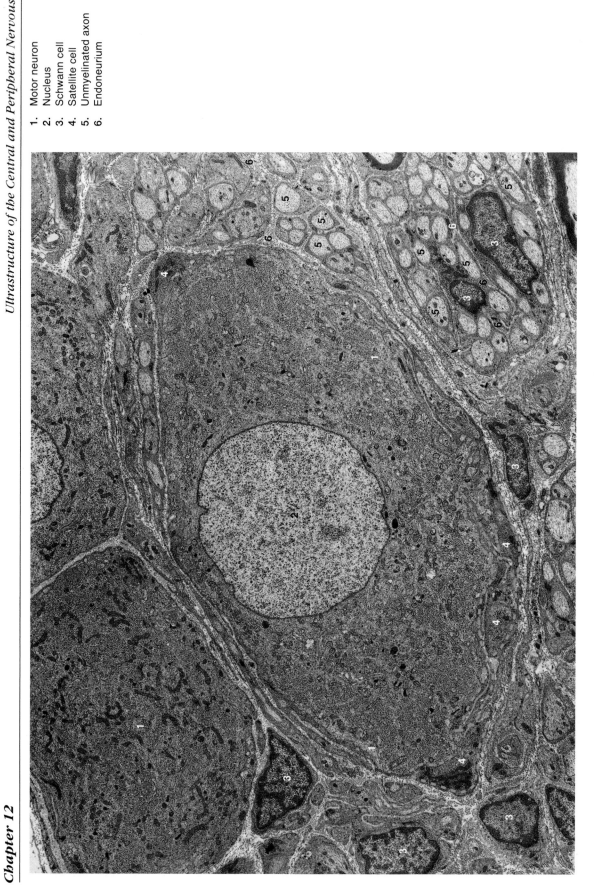

FIGURE 12-9.

Multipolar ganglion cells of the autonomic nervous system (paracervical ganglion).

Chapter 12

1. Unmyelinated axon
2. Unmyelinated nerve fiber
3. Endoneurium
4. Perineurium
5. Fibroblast
6. Neuro-endocrine SIF (**S**mall **I**ntensely **F**luorescing) ganglion cell

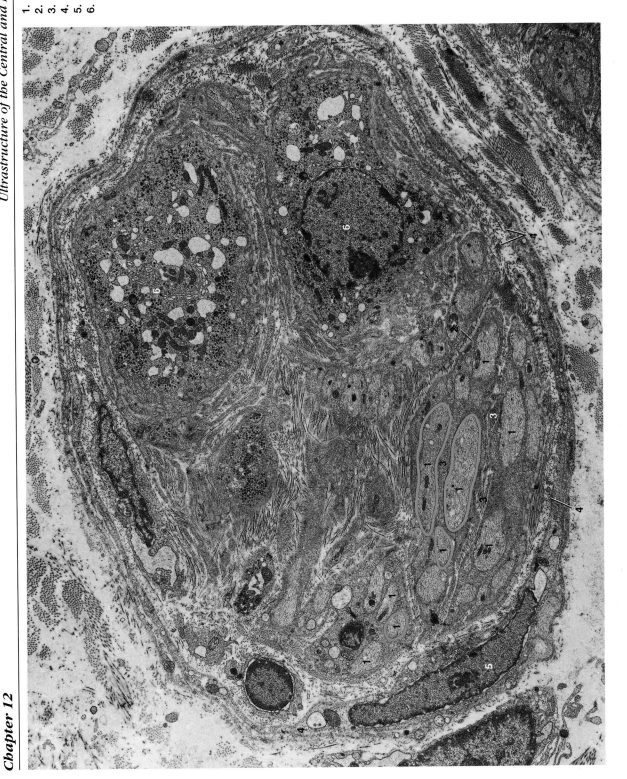

FIGURE 12-10.
Peripheral nerve bundle and ganglion of the autonomic nervous system.

Ultrastructure of the Central and Peripheral Nervous Systems

1. Axoplasm
2. Neurotubules
3. Neurofilaments
4. Myelin
5. Internal mesaxon
6. External mesaxon
7. Axolemma
8. Mitochondrium
9. Endoneurium
10. Cytoplasm of Schwann cell
11. Nucleus of Schwann cell
12. Unmyelinated nerve fiber

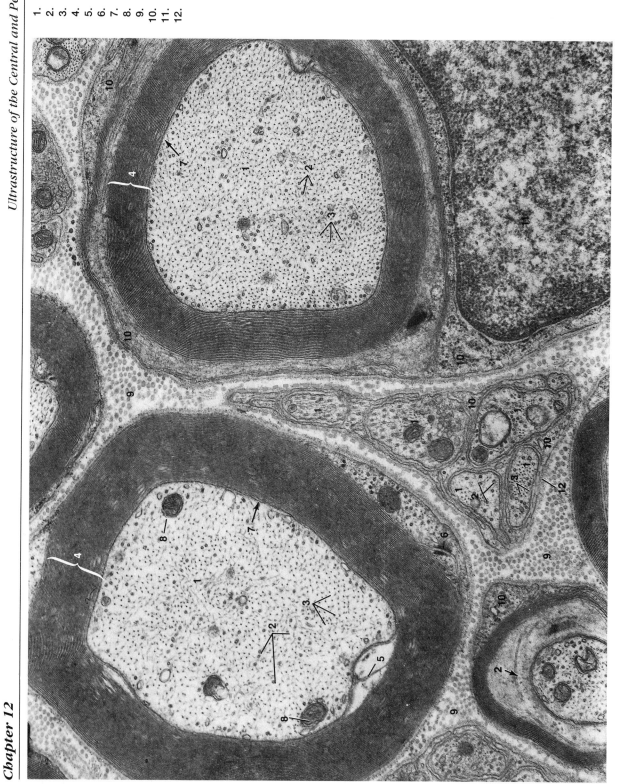

FIGURE 12-11.
Nerve fiber of the peripheral nervous system.

1. Nerve fiber
2. Unmyelinated axon
   (longitudinal section)
3. Dense core vesicles
4. Fibroblast
5. Collagen (perineurium)

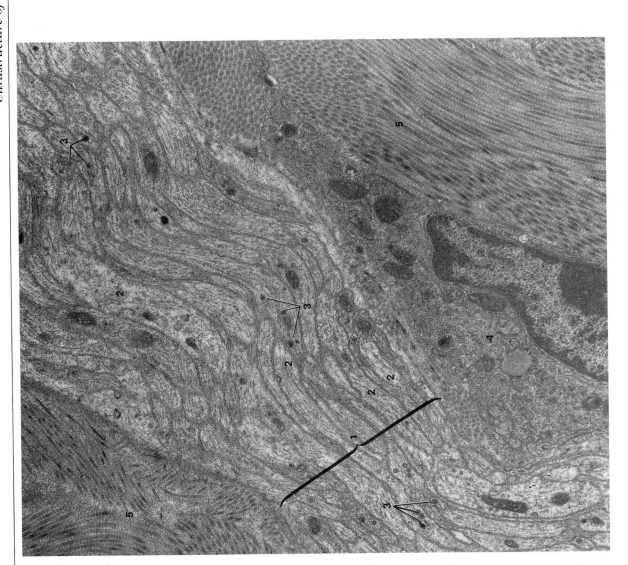

FIGURE 12-12.
Nerve fibers of the autonomic nervous system (intestine).

1. Nerve fiber
2. Unmyelinated axon
3. Nucleus of a smooth muscle cell
4. Cytoplasm of a smooth muscle cell
5. Mitochondrium

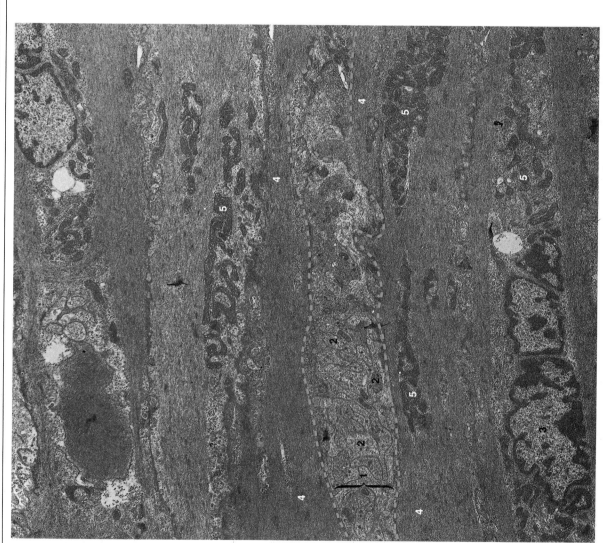

FIGURE 12-13.

Parasympathetic nerve in the muscularis of the intestine.

Index

Boldface numbers indicate the pages on which the main or most illustrative examples are located.